Flower Essences
for Animals

Flower Essences for Animals
Remedies for Helping the Pets You Love

Lila Devi

BEYOND
WORDS
Publishing
I N C

Beyond Words Publishing, Inc.
20827 N.W. Cornell Road, Suite 500
Hillsboro, Oregon 97124-9808
503-531-8700
1-800-284-9673

This book is a reference work not intended to treat, diagnose, or prescribe. The information contained herein is in no way considered as a replacement for consultation
with a duly licensed healthcare professional.

Managing editor: Kathy Matthews
Proofreader: Marvin Moore
Design: Principia Graphica and Dorral Lukas
Composition: William H. Brunson Typography Services

Printed in the United States of America
Distributed to the book trade by Publishers Group West

Library of Congress Cataloging-in-Publication Data
Devi, Lila, date
    Flower essences for animals : remedies for helping the pets you love / Lila Devi.
      p. cm.
    Includes bibliographical references (p.).
    ISBN 1-58270-039-7 (pbk)
    1. Alternative veterinary medicine.   2. Pets—Diseases—Alternative treatment.
  3. Pets—Health.   4. Flowers—Therapeutic use. I. Title.
    SF745.5 .D48   2000
    636.089′55—dc21

                                                              00-063075

The corporate mission of Beyond Words Publishing, Inc.:
    Inspire to Integrity

To Ambrosia and Princess

Anything will give up its secrets if you love it enough.
Dr. George Washington Carver

CONTENTS

FOREWORD

During my years in private practice, I have utilized the combined resources of excellent medical training received at the University of California, Davis School of Veterinary Medicine, and my study of acupuncture and traditional Chinese medicine. Even before I became a veterinarian, I sought holistic care for my family animals. I realized that there must be ways to invoke healing other than with drugs, many of which suppress the immune system in their effort to rid the patient of debilitating or annoying symptoms. Now, as a practitioner, I am certain that natural methods of healing often have greater benefits than the modern medicine options consisting primarily of synthetic drug therapy and surgery.

Alternative veterinarians, those who use various disciplines outside of conventional medicine—examples being homeopathy, herbals, chiropractic, acupuncture, and flower essences—have been inspired by the positive results. Cases that were either not resolved by or have become refractory to the usual medical protocols are often referred to us. An example follows.

A four-year-old miniature dachshund was referred to our clinic with a fluid-filled abdomen from severe chronic liver disease. She arrived with one week's worth of medication, since it was believed she would not even live that long. The referring veterinarian, an internal medicine specialist, felt she had exhausted all that modern medicine could provide and that any hope would lie in a different approach. For me, the hope for survival was in this little dog's eyes. She was willing to keep trying. So, we did acupuncture to access Qi and activate the healing ability that God provides in every life form. I prescribed Chinese herbs known to soothe the liver and restore normal function. Flower essences were added to her drinking water to maintain a positive attitude. Within one month, she had regained her normal size and returned to her usual dominant, opinionated self, ruling the household. It is now over a year later and she continues to live a happy, excellent-quality life. Presently, she is on flower essences to keep her from being too bossy!

Another common challenge is the companion with a behavioral imbalance. These animals are typically passed on to unsuspecting new families or destroyed. The use of flower essences has not only made a great difference in how these individuals respond but has provided a road map into understanding their emotional makeup. One case follows. A two-dog household had suffered destruction and despair when, coming home from work, their humans discovered the aftermath of their fighting. Attempts were made to keep them apart, either in separate rooms or even one inside and the other outside. Coming home to carpet and doors chewed beyond repair and windows broken, the humans were about to give up but could not decide which dog was to leave. They decided instead to try flower essences prescribed by an animal communicator, adjusted every couple months as the dogs changed their attitudes about themselves, each other, and where they wanted to live. Now this family lives in harmony.

Often, viewing our animal friends through an emotional light and treating them accordingly has the benefit of healing many of the physical manifestations as well. Linking mental health with physical health is not a new concept, and it is in fact the basis for flower essence treatment. Observe and analyze the animal's emotional state, administer a flower remedy, and watch the restoration of health on all levels.

Each living thing has a life-force energy; it resonates and is complete. When subjected to the stresses of everyday living, parts of our essence are diminished and leave us out of sorts. Animals are no different. Our domesticated animal companions are now limited to what we provide for them and can no longer forage for what they need in the wild. Cats and dogs, for example, eat grass when they feel a need to purge themselves. Though ancestrally tinctures may not have been the mode of introduction, so many cultures around the world have passed down their understanding and observations of how plants impart healing. And whereas animals used to be able to dose themselves on wild plants, now we can do the same for them with flower essence tinctures. Flower essence therapy is a sophisticated, subtle, effective way to glean nature's healing power.

Lila Devi has presented a thorough, well-researched guide to using flower essences for balancing and healing effects. Lila shares not only her extensive knowledge of applying flower essence therapy but also her embracing love for the animal kingdom. I encourage anyone looking for more natural means of healing to incorporate the wisdom expressed in the following pages.

Rena Ferreira, D.V.M
Sierra Animal Wellness Center
Gold Run, California

ACKNOWLEDGMENTS

With gratitude to the animals for the beauty, depth, and laughter they bring into our lives. Thank you for sharing your secrets.

Special thanks to Rena Ferreira, D.V.M.; Cathy Parojinog; Dr. Peter Van Houten; Dr. David Kessler; John Novak; the staff at Beyond Words Publishing; Jeanie Alonzi; Sonia Fitzpatrick; John Helin; Tim Tschantz; Karen LoCicero; Anna Drummond; J. Donald Walters; Paramhansa Yogananda; my husband, Doug Stone; the veterinarians, animal lovers, and pet owners who have contributed their stories; and the bobcat who won our staring contest fifteen feet outside my back door.

INTRODUCTION

I once saw a cartoon depicting two terriers strolling down a lane, one saying to the other, "Why is it always 'Sit,' 'Fetch,' 'Roll over,' and never 'Think,' 'Discriminate,' 'Be yourself'?" Our animal friends, clever and entertaining in their own ways, deserve our loving care and support. When we remove them from their natural habitats in the wild and domesticate them as pets, it becomes our responsibility to provide them with the best care possible. In return, they enhance our lives. Studies have shown that pet owners live happier, healthier, and even longer lives than non–pet owners. Our job in caring for our animal friends may be great, but our rewards are indeed many.

Flower essences—herbal tinctures for strength and balance—are a wonderful means of natural pet care. They address a wide range of psychological and emotional issues for animals and people alike. Subtle, yes; weak, no. In gentle, non-invasive ways, they provide a "taste of nature" in a language at once familiar and accessible to animals. Since its inception in 1977, my company, Master's Flower Essences, has been the recipient of testimonials from pet owners and animal lovers worldwide. Flower essences have enriched not only their pets' lives but their own as well.

I would like to propose a new meaning for the word *pet* to replace the standard dictionary definition, "an animal kept for amusement or companionship." Although animals can entertain us endlessly, this definition diminishes their stature and subtly implies that they exist primarily for our own sport. Based on a secondary dictionary definition—"one especially cherished or indulged"—I suggest the following: "A pet is an animal whom we domesticate in exchange for providing the highest possible quality of care." In this sense, it is we who are subservient, we who are the servants.

As for the word *owner* in this context, to imply that pets belong to us is an accurate statement, but to think that we possess them because we have paid for them as though they were property does not do justice to our role. Here, too, I propose a new definition for the word *owner* as it applies to animals and pets: that we own the responsibility for their care, with a lifetime commitment. And through their dearness and innocence, is it not they who own us?

Now we come to the somewhat awkward grammatical issue of gender: Is a pet a *he*, a *she*, or an *it*? Referring to a pet as an "it" is, to me, unthinkable. Though I by no means consider myself a chauvinist, I will refer to a singular pet, animal, and occasional person by the commonly used masculine pronoun, *he*, for the sake of simplicity. Also, I will use the relative pronoun *who* rather than *that*. In addition, I will use the masculine pronouns *he* and *his* for pet owners for the sake of clarity rather than switching back and forth from masculine to feminine, which can be somewhat confusing. I sincerely hope that the reader will not take offense at this usage of the English language.

It is common these days to find veterinarians who work with herbs or homeopathy. Flower essences, too, are making their way into mainstream pet care. Oftentimes immediately, animals respond to them. Some of our most enthusiastic customers are gift, health, and pet stores that cater to the needs of pet owners and animal lovers. Well over half the households in America now have pets. An estimated 59 million cats and 54 million dogs, plus 12 million fish and over 7 million reptiles, inhabit homes in the United States. Our office receives regular testimonials about cats, dogs, horses, rabbits, ferrets, fish, and birds, as well as other animals both domesticated and in the wild, whose lives are significantly improved through flower essences. In fact, many animals whose behaviors or health problems were so severe that they were destined for euthanasia have been helped and enabled to live out their lives. Although this book offers many stories about cats and dogs, the twenty essences described herein apply to any species or breed. Fear, loneliness, and trauma are common experiences for all animals, including humans. From ants to antelopes and emus to elephants, we're all basically the same when it comes to common shared experiences and emotional states. We will, however, experience them to varying degrees according to our level of consciousness, as I discuss in chapter 1.

Healing with flowers is not new. Throughout time, fine-tuned survival instincts have led animals to graze on plants for their restorative properties. Animals know when to abstain from food to cleanse and restore their digestive systems; they understand when it is time to withdraw, lay low, and sleep to regenerate their bodies; and they sense when to walk off into the woods to die. Flower essences parallel and support their ancient wisdom.

Indeed, it is we who have sacrificed balanced living at the feet of our own self-created stress and lack of connection with natural living and Mother Nature, carrying domesticated animals along in our wake. Through their nobility and purity, abundantly given in their unconditional friendships with us, we may re-establish a healthy communion with all living things. *Flower Essences for Animals* is offered to help us, as custodians of our animal friends, to provide them with the most sensitive and effective care possible through the practical application of flower essences.

Keyword Qualities
of the
Master's Flower Essences

Almond	Self-control
Apple	Healthfulness
Avocado	Good memory
Banana	Humility
Blackberry	Purity
Cherry	Cheerfulness
Coconut	Upliftment
Corn	Vitality
Date	Sweetness, tenderness
Fig	Flexibility
Grape	Love, devotion
Lettuce	Calmness
Orange	Joy
Peach	Selflessness
Pear	Peacefulness
Pineapple	Self-assuredness
Raspberry	Kindheartedness
Spinach	Simplicity
Strawberry	Dignity
Tomato	Strength, courage

1
THE ANIMAL KINGDOM:
A THINKING, FEELING, CONSCIOUS DOMAIN

Animals are sleeping immortals.
Paramhansa Yogananda

Have you ever had your day brightened by seeing a dog enjoy a car ride, his head lolling out the window of a passing vehicle, the wind ruffling his fur? Or in the way your cat greets you after work, her tail tip twitching to beat the band in the excitement of welcoming you home? How about when your pet ferret somersaults across the floor, backflips off the sofa, ricochets off the wall, and then does it all over again just for fun? These tiniest of gestures, communicating a myriad of meanings, can make our day or even change our lives.

We love our animal friends. We love to see them happy, healthy, chipper, and spunky. We ache when they hurt. We care for them. And in that care, we have many choices. This is a book about one such option: flower essences for animals.

Flower essences may be called "metaphysical herbs," or herbs that work on a beyond-the-physical level. In contrast, allopathic medications, from prescription to over-the-counter drugs, work biochemically. Western medicines exert their effect by specifically or nonspecifically reversing or neutralizing the symptoms of a physiological process gone awry. For example, if a person eats incorrectly, he may develop an ulcer, creating a biochemical problem. Scientists have learned ways to prevent the cells of the stomach from secreting excessive amounts of acid, which will in turn allow it to heal. We see here a specific biochemical blockade or enhancement to alleviate the ulceration and its physical causes.

Flower essences, on the other hand, work on the spiritual or psychological state underlying the physical condition; they do not need to pass through the digestive system for absorption. They address the problem at the level of thought or emotion that precedes the physical disharmony. Since not all people who eat incorrectly will develop ulcers, the question arises as to why some people develop this condition and others do not. Essential flower essence philosophy suggests treating the deeper cause, balancing the personality so that the individual may heal himself.

Many people today, including some in the medical profession, are recognizing the importance of treating the root cause of physical disorders rather than the resultant symptoms. Dr. John Lee of Mill Valley, California, who recently retired from forty years of medical practice, says that we are "collecting patients from the wrong end of the river." In other words, people would arrive at his office asking to have their strokes, heart attacks, and cataracts "fixed" rather than discovering and remedying what caused them to become ill in the first place. He observed that people made wrong life choices that eventually caused discomfort, if not life-threatening illnesses.

In our role as pet owners, we can make choices concerning the care of our pets. (Note: For a new definition of *pets* and *pet owners*, please see the introduction to this book.) Flower essences, a truly holistic form of natural pet care, affect energy and heighten awareness. Since 1977, I have collected countless testimonies confirming that flower essences are especially helpful for animals, simply because their natures are far less complicated than those of human beings, and thus the natural effects of the essences are significantly less blocked or constricted. To summarize, their personalities don't get in the way.

Also, we find that the placebo effect is simply not an issue for animals. We may define the placebo phenomenon as a therapeutic benefit obtained from a substance, procedure, or activity that, in and of itself, should not have any effect and, for most people, would be completely noneffective. This dynamic seems to be mediated in ways that we do not completely understand, but we do know that a person's belief that it will work dramatically improves the odds that it does work. It is not unusual in medication trials, for example, to find a blood-pressure drug that tests at 60 percent effectiveness, while 25 to 35 percent of the placebo-taking subjects also show improvements. In people, the placebo effect is accountably strong.

So potent are placebo results that they are recognized and respected by the medical profession. According to Dr. Peter Van Houten, a medical doctor in family practice in Nevada City, California, "In giving a medication for the first time, a wise physician will affirm to his patients that it will work well without problems. This approach augments the ability of the medicine to provide the desired result." Animals, on the other hand, do not conjure up results as do people; the placebo effect, for them, is inoperative. When a flower essence works, behavioral changes are noted; if it doesn't work, symptoms remain the same.

These examples illustrate a point that is both commonplace and fascinating: animals are different from human beings. They intrigue, baffle, and amuse us. It is helpful, therefore, in the context of a book about improved care for them, to understand the animals' level of awareness and also their particular placement in the grander scheme of this world. Through working with their unique personalities, traits, and behaviors, we can then know how to effectively administer flower essences for their well-being.

A Context for Understanding Animals

The East Indian rishis—sages throughout time, or "living textbooks" of ancient truths—have explained the evolution of consciousness through the mineral, plant, and animal kingdoms as follows: "God sleeps in the minerals, dreams and cries in the plants, begins to stir in the animals, and is capable of fully awakening in humanity." This portrait of the evolution of consciousness is further explained in terms of five sheaths, or veils— *koshas*, in Sanskrit—that dull the faculty of awareness in all living things. Through a gradual process, as each sheath falls away a higher level of awareness emerges.

The mineral kingdom of inorganic matter, including rocks and precious gems, is encased in all five *koshas*. The fifth is the *annamaya kosha*, or matter sheath. We might remember the "pet rock" companion inundating the toy market some years back. The rock was an easy-to-care-for pet—no feeding, no cleaning—but, alas, not much awareness. Members of the mineral kingdom—crystalline in color, structure, and hardness—compose this least-evolved group of living things. Life sleeps in this kingdom.

However, the mineral kingdom does possess some awareness. Metal fatigue—and the fact that metal possesses some level of consciousness—is now an acknowledged phenomenon. In my first book, *The Essential Flower Essence Handbook*, I have documented some of the findings of the Indian botanist Dr. Jagadis Chandra Bose, who developed instruments for measuring the response of metals to various stimuli.

When the "matter" sheath dissolves through the evolutionary process, we find the plant kingdom emerging, exposing the life sheath, or *pranamaya kosha*. Here, life expresses itself through the beauty and form of plants, characterized by cellulose cell walls and growth through synthesis of inorganic substances. A primary, distinguishing factor of the plant kingdom, as we shall later see, is its lack of locomotive skills. Thus, life dreams in this kingdom.

Yet plants can communicate with other living beings, including with each other. Trees, by way of example, are conscious that they are alive and make an effort to protect and preserve themselves. One particular kind of tree, if attacked by a certain leaf mold, will send a warning message to other neighboring trees, who then produce a chemical within their systems that filters into their leaves and prevents the mold from growing.

Next, the mind sheath, or *manomaya kosha*, falls away, revealing the animal kingdom. Webster defines an animal as "any organism of the kingdom animalia, distinguished from plants by certain typical characteristics, such as the power of locomotion, fixed structure and limited growth, and non-photosynthetic metabolism." Animals possess the power of movement, which enables them the benefit of accessing different localities. The sheer joy of animals at play—jumping, climbing, racing, diving—is a clear expression of their exploration of the freedom of movement. Within ten minutes after his birth, a goat kid is standing on spindly legs; a few days later, he is frolicking on cliffs and crags. Although plants may be transported as their seeds are windborne—the dandelion, for example—it is the combination of the ability to direct their own movement and being aware that allows animals to perceive and learn through covering greater territory. And so, in the animal kingdom, life stirs and further awakens.

Thus, we see an evolution of consciousness from one kingdom to the next as the *koshas*, or veils that dull awareness, are removed. Without suggesting that one is more valuable than the other, most people would agree that a dog is more aware than a sea slug. Life's delightful beauty lies in its infinite variety of expression. The leopard's spots and the zebra's stripes are proof of a supremely conscious design and Designer both! The point is that a universal and innate drive exists in all living beings to increase their aware-ness. All life forms express this desire.

The *jnanamaya kosha*, or the discriminative sheath, is then exposed, and mankind enters the picture. In humans, the intellect has developed to a level of discrimination, thought, and reason. It is on this level that life, in the form of man, gains the element of will, and thus free choice. We may use our thoughts and actions positively, to evolve, or negatively, to close ourselves down to greater awareness. Herein lies the potential pitfall for all human beings: The major disadvantage of free will is that we can choose to think or behave in ways that act contrary to our best interest.

Overeating is a prime example. Injurious to the body and mind alike, we go for that second helping. Through misuse of reason and abandonment of common sense, we demonstrate our lack of attunement with nature's wisdom. On the other hand, one never sees overweight animals in the wild. (A growing problem, in fact, is obesity in domesticated animals as we bring them into environments that are removed from nature and thus unnatural to them.)

Animals do not possess the element of choice inherent in free will. Since they do not have the ability to make wrong choices, they are incapable of mankind's foibles; self-aggrandizement does not exist in the animal kingdom. It is for this very reason, one suspects, that people are so drawn to animals: We recognize their lack of ego, the "inner Eden" state to which we ourselves wish to return. In this sense, they possess a purity and innocence that humans often lack. A life lived in harmony with nature radiates an innate beauty and spiritu-ality, reflective of Nature herself. At the same time, because of their ability to use reason and make choices, human beings are far less driven and controlled by their instinctive nature than animals.

Another interesting distinction between man and the lower animals is that adultery, as we know it, does not exist in the animal kingdom. Even though their behavior with multiple partners may seem indiscriminate to us, sex for them is purely an act of procreation to propagate the species. It harbors no moral issues. Nor is divorce a subject of concern for them—including legal fees and child support. The bonobo, a pigmy chimpanzee of which less than twenty thousand remain in Zaire, are as close as it comes to an exception. This recently discovered breed appears to use the sex act not only as an alternative to confrontational behavior and to calm their rivalry over food but also for pleasure. Although apes can sometimes be trained to have the intelligence of a human child, we may surmise that the bonobo behavior lacks the maturity and discrimination usually seen in adult humans.

As a human being evolves, the final sheath, the bliss sheath, or *anandamaya kosha*, falls away, and the state of Self-realization described in every major religion is achieved. Through right use of the quality of free choice, one experiences the state of nondualistic ecstasy and thus awakens fully.

Anatomical Insights: The Brain

In scientific terms, this concept of evolution can be explained through a basic study of the brain. When we look at man and most of the vertebrate animals, such as reptiles, birds, and mammals, we find that they possess an area of the brain called the limbic system, so named because it is anatomically shaped like a half moon. This area, deep inside the brain, is fairly similar in a cat, a rabbit, and a man. In all creatures it performs a similar function—even in reptiles, who are more simple and primitive than mammals.

In man and other animals, the limbic system is the area of the brain concerned with instinctual functions and basic behaviors, such as rage and fear. Examples of limbic function at work may be seen in a junkyard dog's ferocity in defending its territory or an animal's panic when attacked by larger, more aggressive animals. Behaviors attributed to the limbic system include the preservation of self as well as the instinct to reproduce. These behaviors apply to man as well. In human beings, the limbic system functions as a built-in, instinctual safety net.

What separates us from other animals is the degree to which our prefrontal lobes—the seat of the intellect—are developed. This area of the brain is the key that ultimately distinguishes us from lower animals—although other structural differences exist in the brain, obviously, between us and gorillas or rabbits. In a few of the animals, such as dolphins, prefrontal lobe capabilities exist, though in very limited ways.

The prefrontal lobes of the brain are the most anterior portion of the frontal lobes, located directly behind the forehead and between the eyebrows. It is that area of the brain which is concerned with our power of concentration; our level of happiness and well-being; certain aspects of creativity; our ability to learn new things; our willpower and our willingness to stick with a specific task; our ability to extract generalities from assimilated information; and, perhaps most importantly, our idealism and aspirations.

The interesting thing is that in man the prefrontal lobes actually exert an inhibitory effect on the limbic system, essentially acting as an override mechanism. This is what we see in longtime meditators: a quieting of the limbic system occurs, automatically inhibiting the more primitive, instinctual behaviors driven by this function of the brain.

In meditation, the focus of the brain's function shifts to the prefrontal lobes, the part that distinguishes us from other animals. Thus the brain and nervous system are positively affected in the meditator. Physiologically, the overall effect of meditation can be described as a relaxation response, in which the "relax and repose" portion of the central nervous system is emphasized over the "fight or flight" portion. Both during and following meditation, people exhibit lowered pulse rates, lower blood pressure, and better functioning of their organs of regeneration, such as the liver, kidneys, and intestines. Also present is a dramatic decrease in the secretion of stress hormones, such as adrenaline and cortisone.

While it is true that every kind thought a person thinks will raise his energy and increase his awareness that all living things are a part of his own greater reality, the practice of meditation can hasten this process. Scientific studies have shown that meditation improves self-esteem, gives a broader worldview, makes one less self-involved, and reduces neurotic behaviors and psychological annoyances, such as anxiety and depression.

Pain: Animal versus Human

Although some people may argue that a stalk of broccoli has feelings too, including the ability to feel pain, most would agree that a cow has appreciably more advanced feelings than a green cruciferous vegetable. We would also concur that a horse is far more aware than a terrestrial gastropod mollusk, commonly known as a slug. This explanation harbors no judgment; rather, it fosters respect for life in all forms. Some Eastern religious followers, in fact, go to great length to avoid stepping on the tiniest insects as they stroll.

The pain, rage, and terror that animals experience in being led to their death at slaughterhouses is virtually unimaginable. If, however, a group of people were led into a room and told that they would be killed, their suffering would far exceed that of the animals. The people's agony in this identical situation would be multiplied to an intolerable level. Metaphysically encased in one remaining *kosha*, represented by prefrontal lobe capability, humans would possess an even greater awareness of their situation.

Animals deal directly with pain in the moment they experience it. They do what they have to do to avoid it, if possible, or to adapt to it. One "animal communicator"—a person who can communicate telepathically with animals—attended an elderly black Lab suffering from severe arthritis and reported, "This dog just goes and goes. It's not an issue for him; he simply deals with it. His attitude seems to be that this is the way it is, and he'll try to get comfortable."

Animals suffer physical pain due to the stimulation of the nerves. A fox with its leg caught in a trap, for example, would feel the pain of the clamp and tearing of the flesh with a full nervous-system response. A human being in that same situation would suffer the additional agony of mental anguish: "What if I lose the leg, how will I support my family? What about my job? Is this covered by my insurance? How will I get by in the future?" and so on. Thus, a person experiences a much greater component of suffering than the physical response alone. Animals live in the moment, accepting what happens and dealing with it at the time, unlike we who often live simultaneously in the past and future. In this way, we could say that they deal with pain better than we do. Plus, they don't take it so personally. Our identification with our body, and the resultant thought that this is *my* leg and *my* pain, increases the suffering many times over.

Instinct versus Intuition

As mentioned earlier, animals do not have free choice, generally speaking, as does mankind. Instinct and nature, rather than free will, are their guides as they remain encased in the third *kosha*. Some animals form pair bonds; others live in packs. Some animals are altruistic—they will sacrifice their lives for their partners or their families, whether an animal group or a human household.

The current scientific mode of thought is to observe each behavior of an animal and analyze it according to whether it increases or decreases the possibility of the perpetuation of genes of that particular animal or its species. It inquires: Can that animal reproduce? If a wolf confronts a moose charging his pack, is the wolf bravely altruistic for laying down his life so that the pack may survive the encounter? This particular school of animal behavior would say that, based on statistical evidence, the wolf's actions are a specific display of cunning to allow the pack's continued existence. Thus the gene pool is perpetuated. In this light, the wolf's behavior is not altruistic, even though it appears so. It is instinct.

One expression of instinct, it might be said, is an inherent, nature-based form of altruism. If a dog saves his household from a fire (see chapter 3), what is his fundamental, motivating instinct? Preservation, or continued existence. In addition, the dog wants to preserve the bond and relationship with his human family. Animals grieve when their loved ones—of their own species or others—are lost. Their lament transcends the realm of instinct.

When a pet crosses the line between instinct and intuition, extraordinary, extrasensory events happen. Some time ago, I read of a married couple who had to relocate to the state of Washington from Minnesota, regretfully leaving their cat behind in the care of neighbors. Six months and fourteen hundred or more miles later, the cat walked up their driveway. Was that cat's action based on instinct—or love?

Many documented cases of animals tending to humans have recently come to light. One such story originates in Belgium at a therapeutic riding center for autistic children. Horses usually become spooked with anyone walking under their bellies, but here they remained placidly accommodating. Behaviors such as sudden outbursts by the children would normally cause the horses to rear, kick, and eventually flee, but here they were uncharacteristically calm instead. This story illustrates the horses' ability to override their natural instincts with altruistic actions.

Recently, a large school of dolphins was beached off the coast of Florida. Bottlenose dolphins usually remain fifty to sixty miles from the coast, but some had caught infections and were very ill. The healthy dolphins remained with the ill, unable to break themselves away from the cries of the failing ones. Whether we anthropomorphize their behavior or not, this story illustrates a beautiful aspect of the bond that living beings feel for one another. In hearing tales of such uplifting nobility, the controversy over projecting human characteristics onto animals falls aside. In a very human way, they are willing to sacrifice themselves to keep others alive. And we are touched.

Wild animals must depend on their own skills, and perhaps those of a partner or pack, to ensure their survival. Everyone else is a threat until they prove themselves otherwise. When we domesticate animals, we cross a boundary of trust and interaction. We silently communicate that they no longer need to live by survival instincts, that we will feed and shelter them. Herein lies a beautiful gift: The animal extends his sense of group trust and identification to include the human family. And this behavior is noble, whether it stems from instinct or not.

In Conclusion

Animals and saints—on either side of the free-choice maelstrom, in terms of evolution of consciousness—share one trait, especially, in common. They love us unconditionally. And for this reason, we can't help but love them in return. "Everybody loves a lover," as the saying goes, which accurately defines the nature of our animal companions. Our pets love us without condition; and in this respect, they are often more advanced than their owners. They love us above and beyond the level of personality and its resultant behavior: whether we are good or bad, punctual or procrastinating, tidy or sloppy.

In many ways, we could say that animals are more spiritual than we are. We see unbridled delight in the eyes of their newborn, a challenging playfulness in the bodies of their young, and a maturing wisdom in the graceful form of their elders. Nature is their native country; natural rhythms are their language. Animals are extrasensorially perceptive. They live each moment with unbounded fullness. They give themselves to life, holding back nothing, abandoning all barriers. They love readily and completely.

Is it any wonder, then, that animals are our teachers?

2

FLOWER ESSENCES AND HOW THEY WORK

The soil, in return for her service, keeps the tree tied to her;
the sky asks nothing and leaves it free.
Rabindranath Tagore

We may credit Welsh doctor Edward Bach, who left his medical practice in London in 1930, with the discovery of flower essences, or flower remedies as they are sometimes called. Seeking an inexpensive and painless means of curing his patients, Dr. Bach evolved a simple healing approach over the next six years that addressed their mental and emotional states rather than treating their physical symptoms. He was a truly holistic doctor, ahead of his time. Correct the psychological state, he reasoned, and the physical body stands a better chance of overcoming its ailments.

Employing Bach's method of preparation, I developed the Master's Flower Essences in 1977, the second oldest essence line in the world today. These essences were initially interpreted by an internationally renowned teacher from India named Paramhansa Yogananda. He asserted that fresh fruits and vegetables heal us on psychological as well as nutritional levels. Eat cherries for cheerfulness, he recommended, and pears for their peacefulness. These definitions have provided the cornerstone for the twenty Master's Flower Essences, extracted from the blossoms of organic fruit trees and vegetable plants.

Flower essences are prepared through a simple method employing pure spring water, sunlight, and freshly picked blossoms. The flowers are floated in a plain crystal or glass bowl filled with pure spring water for three to four hours in direct morning sunlight with no interference from clouds. The blossoms are then removed, and the water is stored in a dark bottle to prevent further exposure to sunlight, half filled with brandy as a preservative. This preparation is called *mother essence*. (Stock and Dosage bottle directions follow later in this chapter under "Administering an Essence.")

Easy to use and quick-acting, these essences help restore people, animals, and even other plants to their natural state of balance. Seemingly irreversible negative behaviors can be improved or, more often, completely dissolved. Flower essences are completely safe. There are no such things as overdoses, side effects, or contraindications. In the best-case scenario, "miracles" happen—meaning one is returned to a state of wholeness; in the worst case, there is no noticeable response. Please remember: Flower essences do not directly treat physical ailments, nor are they meant to replace proper medical or veterinary care. They will, however, nurture and support your pet's healing process.

Basically, flower essences reestablish an animal's link with his own natural ability to heal himself. In returning him to a state of equilibrium, flower essences simply allow him to do what comes naturally: to be well again. In treating the underlying cause of the illness, we see the opposite of a vicious cycle: The animal's improved psychological health affects his physical state for the better, and vice versa. Or better yet, flower essences can be used to strengthen the animal to prevent illness in the first place!

Your pet's behavioral imbalances, which flower essences address so directly, are often clues and precursors to physical illness. This is not to say that all emotional imbalances eventually become physical illnesses. Oftentimes, it is enough to treat the animal's obvious unhappiness, uneasiness, or fear so as to avoid any physical expression of these symptoms at a later time. As we know, we ourselves are far more likely to be well when we live relatively stress-free, harmonious, and loving lives.

What, then, are the mental and emotional states that affect an animal's wellness? This is the special focus of *Flower Essences for Animals*. Many common pet issues are addressed in this book, with recommendations for remedies, including Pear Essence, to restore stability, security, and equilibrium; Grape Essence, for loneliness, abandonment, jealousy, and the time of a pet's passing; Spinach Essence, for the various stresses of domesticated life, for abuse, especially for strays, and for premature weaning; and Tomato Essence, for the many fears that animals (and we as well) may experience. Flower essences have been proven through countless case histories and testimonials to foster happy and healthy animals and our richly rewarding relationships with them. (Please note: The capitalized plant or food refers to the flower essence, to distinguish it from the food source.)

Animals in Our Lives

Consider these stories. A cat, hearing a burglar breaking into the house at 2 A.M., awakens her owner, who then turns on the light, scaring off the thief. A dog sits by the window every evening, precisely ten minutes before his owner's arrival home, even though the man's work schedule is completely irregular. A gorilla in a Chicago zoo makes front-page news for carrying to safety a stunned child who had fallen over a railing and had plummeted two stories down a concrete cliff into a pit below. On video for all the world to see, an amateur photographer filmed the young gorilla mother gathering up the unconscious three-year-old boy. Not only did she protect the boy from other gorillas as she knuckle-walked him to safety, but she then gently laid him down near the cage door where the zookeepers could safely retrieve him.

Animals actively participate in our lives. They make wonderful companions, seeing us through our most joyful and difficult life experiences. They share our homes day after day. They befriend us through illness and surgery; they comfort us through loss of family and friends. They weather our moves, our moods, our gains and losses alike. Our pets never criticize or judge; nor do they blame or belittle. And through it all, they transform us.

I am often asked by pet owners how they can better care for their animal friends. Perhaps the dog is recovering from surgery or the cat seems unsettled by the sudden return of the children from summer vacation. A vast range of your pet's symptoms and behaviors are easily addressed through the wise use of flower essences. This chapter will supply you with the basic information about how and when to administer essences to your pet.

How Flower Essences Work

Flower essences can be used to help an unwell animal return to health or to assist a happy, well-adjusted animal in feeling even better. Here are just a few examples of the successful use of flower essences for an animal's behavioral problems. An older cat is given an essence and recovers three times more quickly from surgery. A finicky dog calms down and returns to eating regular meals. A newborn goat kid who exhibits symptoms of not surviving through the night— listless, stunned, and disinterested in nursing—spends his first night indoors receiving an essence dosage every half hour and returns to his mother "on all fours" by morning. Another newborn goat kid is brought back to life by an essence after a warm comfrey bath had failed.

Behavioral as well as physiological problems respond to flower essences. A six-year-old cat who had been abandoned as a kitten behaves in a less needy manner, according to his owner, after only two days on an essence program. Another cat immediately stops dominating the other household pets upon being placed on an essence regimen. A pet tortoise, disoriented by an Indian summer change of climate and eating less in preparation for winter hibernation, is noticeably soothed by an essence rubbed under her chin and onto her shell.

Animals on flower essences exhibit radically improved behavior not attributable to any variables other than the essences themselves. They may also heal physically much faster than the normally expected recovery time. We don't find skepticism among the animals—only in their human caretakers. Pets, in fact, respond to essences even more quickly than do people, generally requiring only two weeks on a single essence and often a much shorter time. Nothing makes a believer out of a nonbeliever better than witnessing firsthand a pet's dramatic response to an essence program. Flower essences, according to my company's collected research, work whether we believe in them or not. With animals, the placebo effect is not an issue. Quite simply, people who give essences to their pets see results through behavioral changes.

Stephanie Chalmers, D.V.M., of Santa Rosa, California, reports that, based on her experience, flower essences work immediately: "They help pets and their owners survive the really tough times in specific situations. People really need something for their pets that they can use to help them get through the crisis of the moment, whether it be behavioral problems or skin diseases. And I've seen flower essences work quickly, which makes them very useful."

Veterinarians and other healthcare professionals who use flower essences recommend them for pet owners as well. Animals are sensitive to their owners, and vice versa. Pets, by nature, will both absorb and mirror the emotional climate of their household. Not only is it quite common to see the problems within a household reflected in its pets, but it is both predictable and expected. Especially where emotions or anxieties run out of control, a good veterinarian will recommend an essence program for the owner as well. (Chapters 5 and 6 explain how these remedies may benefit you, the caregiver.) At the risk of repetition, it is important to state that flower essences do not replace proper veterinary care or good nutrition. Many health and behavioral problems can be eliminated simply through an improved diet of fresh, vital foods.

Just as traditional herbal remedies biochemically strengthen our natural defenses and sharpen our body-functioning performance, so flower essences fine-tune us mentally and emotionally, allowing us to experience a higher standard of health and well-being on all levels. When the psychological nature is balanced, the body can relax and, many times, heal itself. This principle applies to people and pets alike. *Flower Essences for Animals* focuses on the specific conditions and situations—emergencies to everyday occurrences—in which your pet may need special care.

Do various species, and different breeds within those species, require different essences to accommodate their different instinctual temperaments? No. Trauma—which calls for Pear Essence—is simply trauma, for people, pets, and even plants. One woman reported adding Pear Essence to the watering can when transplanting an indoor ficus tree. This delicate tree tends to lose most of its leaves during the transplanting process. With its roots soaked in Pear-saturated water before the procedure, not a leaf fell.

Administering an Essence

Flower essences may be administered both orally and topically. The best means of application is the one most agreeable to the animal at the time and circumstance of treatment. One excellent method is to moisten your pet's mouth or gums with a few drops placed on your fingertips, once in the morning and again in the evening. Additional doses several times throughout the day are also required. Some animals enjoy the brandy-preservative taste; others turn their noses up at it. It is not uncommon for pet owners to report that their pets quickly "get used to the taste" and soon thereafter actually begin to enjoy it! (One cat actually sits with her mouth open as her owner drops the dosage into her mouth.) The important factor, whichever method you choose, is for your pet to be dosed *at least* four times daily to ensure best results.

Much like homeopathy, flower essences work best when not given too close to feedings—ten minutes before or one hour after a meal or snack is fine. On the other hand, we receive testimonials of pets exhibiting remarkably quick and thorough results with the essences given through food only. You may try this method if you like; but to be safe, you may want to work in addition with topical application or drops in the water source. This applies to emergency and non-acute situations alike—though for crisis conditions, you may dose every few minutes until results are noticed.

Topical applications are as follows. You may add four drops to a small misting bottle or plant sprayer filled with water to spray on your pet, but only if the procedure is agreeable to him. (Most cats are not at all thrilled with this approach.) You'll need to prepare a fresh solution each morning. This is the easiest and most expedient method when transporting a cat or dog on the car seat next to you. Bedding and cages, including travel carriers and trailers, may also be sprayed with the essence solution. The misting method is so effective and non-invasive that some vets rely on it exclusively.

Or you may add four drops to a small amount of liniment or oil or put it directly on your palm and rub or brush it into fur, flesh, feathers, or scales (for reptiles, not fish). Gently rubbing an essence behind the ears, on the paw pads, or on the abdomen or coat makes for a pleasant experience for your pet. Flower essences can also be added to an animal's drinking water— four drops to a bowl of water or sixteen drops to a watering trough—which should be refilled with fresh water every morning. This approach works best as a backup for other methods since a pet will rarely finish an entire water supply and thus not receive the full dosage.

Topical and oral application are equally effective. We receive many stories of birds who crash into large windows or sliding glass doors and then fall to the ground, stunned and seemingly near death. With doses of Pear applied to their beaks every few minutes, they can then quickly fly off to safety. In fact, pet owners have volunteered countless direct testimonials over the years that our Pear Essence is the most effective flower essence they've ever used.

The Master's Flower Essences are available in Stock Concentrate potency; all twenty are used in the same quantity and frequency. The term *Stock* refers to the level of potency in the preparation of the essence and means that only a minute amount is necessary for results. We prepare the Stock bottles by putting two drops of mother essence in a one-ounce dark bottle filled with brandy. To prepare a Dosage bottle, the third and final level of preparation, simply place two Stock drops in a dark one-ounce bottle, add a tablespoon of brandy as a preservative, and fill the remainder of the bottle with pure spring water. When needed, administer four drops from the Dosage bottle, or use two drops of Stock Concentrate.

The Stock and Dosage bottles will retain their potency for six to ten years if stored out of heat, humidity, and sunlight. Thus, you'll want to be careful not to leave essences in a hot vehicle or on a sunny window ledge. Also, if the dropper should touch your pet or your fingers, it may be sterilized to prevent contamination of the essences by placing it for ten minutes in boiling water with a pinch of sea salt.

Other Helpful Hints

There are never any adverse effects from flower essences; they are virtually risk-free. And if several animals share a watering bowl, bucket, or trough, you may rest assured that no harm is possible. Flower essences can supplement other herbal therapies and allopathic medications without contraindications. In other words, if your dog is on antibiotics and flower essences, there is no conflict. They cannot offset or adversely affect each other. Nor need you ever fear overdosing. It is not possible to administer too much of an essence, although the solution may be wasted.

It is possible, however, to give too little and too infrequently, so be sure to follow directions. Some people feel that because animals respond so readily to flower essences, the dosage rules can be stretched by giving the essence once or twice a day instead of the recommended four times. Indeed, many times results are still noticeable. For some animals, no more than this is required. But to best ensure results, it is advisable to adhere to the standard dosage directions. In addition, such is their potency and purity that the same dosage amount and frequency apply to animals of varying sizes and weights—unless you are treating a herd of elephants!

In addition, dependence or addiction—either physiological or psychological—is virtually impossible with flower essence therapy. This applies to animals and humans alike. As mentioned earlier, flower essences do not need to travel through the digestive system and be absorbed in the bloodstream as do biochemical medications.

How long should you keep your pet on an essence? Continue until you see stabilized results, indicated by his return to regular behavioral patterns. Many pet owners report results as quickly as with the first dosage. One owner called our office recently with the news that she noticed immediate results for all three of her dogs who were each placed on a different essence to address their various needs and personalities. "When I came home last week, they were all attentive before I even opened the bottles. They quieted down and sat there with their ears back. This was not their typical welcome-home greeting for me!"

In fact, it is safe to say that we get more feedback of immediate results with animals than with people. We receive many testimonials of animals who acknowledge that their owners bring the essences home. Much like a person saying, "Ah, I feel better already," our pets can sense that help is on the way. Although results are often immediate—within ten minutes—you will usually see the beginning of a response within three days. Five days to two weeks is the standard framework of time needed for an animal to integrate the necessary behavioral changes when only one essence at a time is administered. In cases of deep-rooted fear or trauma, however, a month-long program may be required. If you do not see results within three days—meaning at least the beginning of changes in behavioral patterns—one of three causes is likely: improper selection, not following dosage directions, or the problem resides in the pet owner and not the pet (see chapter 4).

Is your cat sleeping on her favorite sofa again rather than hiding under the bed after a tooth extraction? Is your dog barking at passersby as usual, having recovered from your son leaving for college? Each animal will respond to and complete an essence program at his own pace—anywhere from a single dosage to two weeks, generally speaking. Flower essences are not meant to be taken indefinitely; use them only until regular, healthy behavior is restored or physical symptoms improve or disappear altogether.

Based on over two decades of research and documented cases, I recommend that you give your pet one essence at a time rather than in combination. We tend to see quicker, more noticeable results with this approach. The obvious benefit with this method is that you will know which essence is working. I have often wondered with the combination approach how one actually knows whether all the essences are helpful or if it is a single "right" essence within that combination which triggers the healing response. However, many people combine three to five remedies with excellent results.

The key is this: If you do not hit on the "right" essence with the single-essence approach, you will need to try a second essence within three days, or half an hour in an emergency. If you are undecided between two or more essences, determine the most predominant and immediate issue at hand, and give the corresponding essence. Yes, your dog can take Pear initially for being hit by a car, for several days to a week, or until you see his behavior returning to normal. Then Tomato can help with residual fears, especially if you catch him shying away from moving vehicles after the accident. And the good news is that, because the Master's Flower Essences is a line of only twenty tinctures, there are fewer to choose from. Fears of any kind may be addressed with Tomato; abandonment or neglect, with Grape. For the beginner and the practicing therapist alike, selection is simplified by fewer essences from which to choose.

Lastly, how to know which essences to give to your pet and in what order? Study the essences described in chapters 5 and 6. Familiarize yourself with the charts in the appendix. Then observe your pet's physical symptoms and behavioral clues. A horse will need Tomato for a fear of being transported. A cat who has been abused by a previous owner will benefit from Grape. If you are undecided, give Pear first. Not only is this a good "first choice essence," but it will allow other definitive symptoms to surface more clearly by helping your pet to return to a more balanced, "readable" state. And in fact, for any pet you bring into your household without knowing his previous history, it is a good idea to give Pear, Grape, and Tomato Essences sequentially, just to "cover all the bases" of his needs. Other essences can be added later or when issues present themselves.

With essences for people, we take into consideration what I call the flower/food connection. This approach explains essence selection in terms of food cravings. People who desire calmness through better self-control may like to snack on almonds. Someone coming to terms with a better sense of self may enjoy a hair shampoo listing strawberry as an ingredient. Although this concept does not apply as readily to animals, we do receive an occasional testimonial in support of the flower/food connection: the elderly dog on Corn Essence who actually enjoys eating corn on the cob, for instance.

For a deeper understanding of the Master's Flower Essences, I refer you to my book, The Essential Flower Essence Handbook. In addition to a full chapter on pets, it provides an in-depth study of each of the twenty essences of this line, mainly for people but also adaptable for animals, as well as other important flower essence information.

In Conclusion

Animals are not skeptical. The multifarious mental blocks that we erect to negate the ways that flower essences work simply do not exist for our pets. One of our most impressive testimonials is of a large tropical fish aquarium being transported from one home to another. When fish are relocated or traumatized in any way, they tend to hide behind their underwater rocks and castles and not surface at feedings for a few days. These angelfish and Jack Dempseys, their tank dosed with a flower essence, exhibited no signs of disturbance; they simply went about their business as usual.

In order to see results with flower remedies, adhering to directions is essential. These bouquets-in-a-bottle can "calm the wild beast" in all living things. One of the more natural herbal supplements available, flower essences balance our pets' lives and our relationships with them as well.

Chapter Summary Outline

1. Dr. Edward Bach discovered flower essences in the 1930s.
2. In 1977, the Master's Flower Essences were developed by Lila Devi based on initial interpretations by Paramhansa Yogananda.
3. The twenty Master's Essences, utilizing fruit and vegetable blossoms, assist us psychologically; their corresponding food sources nourish us physiologically.
4. Flower essences are prepared by a simple method using blossoms, pure spring water, and undisturbed sunlight.
5. The basic philosophy of flower essences is to treat the cause, not the effect. This approach awakens the animal's life force so that he may heal himself.
6. *Flower essences do not replace proper veterinary care or proper nutrition.*
7. Directions: Both oral and topical application are effective. You may choose from the following options:
   a. Moisten your pet's mouth or gums with a few essence drops.
   b. Add four drops to a small misting bottle or plant sprayer filled with water to spray bedding, a room, or a vehicle used for travel.
   c. Add four drops to a fresh water bowl every morning, or sixteen drops to a watering trough.
   d. Add the essence to liniment or oil or directly onto your palm, and rub it on the animal's fur, flesh, feathers, or scales.
8. When to give flower essences:
   a. Not with meals is advised; ten minutes before or one hour after is suggested.
   b. Four times daily is the minimum number of times; more often in emergencies is fine.
9. Other helpful dosage information:
   a. There are no adverse effects.
   b. Animals can share a watering source even if not all of them need the same essence(s).
   c. There are no contraindications or dangers of overdosing.
   d. Following dosage directions, i.e., four times daily, is imperative for effective results.

10. How long to keep your pet on an essence:
    a. Keep your pet on the essence regimen until you see noticeable, stabilized results.
    b. Results generally require five days to two weeks.
    c. If no changes are seen within three days, there are three reasons:
       (1) It may not be the best essence choice.
       (2) Dosage directions are not being properly followed.
       (3) The owner, not the pet, is the cause of the problem.
11. A single-essence program is very effective in treating animals, though combinations of three to five are also successful.
12. Study the twenty essences in order to learn which essence to give and in what order.
    a. Become familiar with the charts in the appendix.
    b. Observe the animal's physical symptoms and behavioral clues.

3
How to Communicate
with Animals

Animals are such agreeable friends—
they ask no questions, they pass no criticisms.
George Eliot

People who talk to plants and hear their responses are noted throughout history, such as George Washington Carver, Luther Burbank, and the brilliant botanist Dr. Chandra Bose (documented in my first book, *The Essential Flower Essence Handbook*). For the most part, however, the different kingdoms of this earth are unable to communicate with each other. Even people and animals, both of the animal kingdom, experience this gap. Basically, people are often clueless in interpreting what their pet's behavior means, unless it is blatant, attention-getting, or even destructive. And yet, to a large extent, animal behavior is completely comprehensible. A deer, by way of example, acts like a deer and not a mountain lion. Or as one sage said, "It is the nature of a fig tree to bear figs."

How can we bridge the communication gap between people and their pets? Our animals talk to us all the time. Many of us speak to them. All that remains is that we silently listen and sensitively hear them. This chapter provides a few techniques to help you develop communication skills with your animal friends—and to better understand how they communicate with us as well. A particular focus is given to dogs, cats, horses, ferrets, rabbits, and birds.

If only communicating with animals could be easily learned from reading a book or taking a seminar! Many animal communicators, psychologists, and behavioral researchers do seem to have a natural gift for relating to animals. Learning to communicate with animals involves a few simple tools presented in this chapter. With a brief look at some species-specific mannerisms, we may begin to relate to their foibles and their charms alike. The following "Politically-Correct Dictionary" for dogs offers a humorous interspecies translation to help us along:

Dog	Domestic partner
Hound	Canine companion
Person	Quadruped-impaired
Pet	Roommate
Master	Master chef
Owner	Automatic door opener
Command	Suggestion
Pot roast	Dog food
Pet groomer	Spa attendant
"Accident"	Self-expression
Barking	Discussing
Discipline	Assertiveness training
Obedience	Self-actualization program
Shedding	Self-renewal
Digging through trash	Recycling
Dog pack	Fraternal organization
Guard dog	Defense chief
Sheep dog	Agricultural management professional
Lap dog	Personal advisor
Stray	Explorer
Kids	Assailants
Bath	Obsolete

The Tools: Listen, Look, and Speak

Listening to animals' voices is one method of "reading" or understanding them. This process is much like learning a foreign language. At first we may hear only a string of strange, unidentifiable sounds. But then we notice the repetition of certain words and phrases. At some point we finally distinguish full sentences complete with various elements of grammar and syntax. In another vein, we can learn to tune in to an animal's state of consciousness like a mother's instinctive attunement to the cries of her child. Within months of his birth, she learns to decipher in her child's cries boredom, discomfort, pain, sadness, fear, frustration, or disorientation.

With some practice, we can learn to hear in the voiced sounds of our animal companions the cry for food, the mating call, an expressed irritation, a call to play. We will "hear" the jealousy of feeling replaced by a newer household pet or the abandonment of being left alone while we have been away on a business trip. These sounds will be further corroborated by the animal's body language: jumping on our lap; bringing us favorite toys or hunted prey; or withdrawing, turning away, refusing food or treats, and so on.

Looking into your pet's eyes—the windows of the soul, as it has been said—is another way of communicating with him. (This method is not advisable with especially fierce dogs, monkeys, or any carnivorous wild animal; they interpret direct eye contact as a confrontation, a threat, or a sign of aggression.) Don't intellectualize your concern for his welfare; *become* that compassion. Don't think love; *become* that love. Animals think in pictures and possess a wealth of emotions, feelings, and intuitive awareness. These are the building blocks of their language.

The owner of Bob Davis, a three-year-old purebred golden retriever, has no problem communicating with him. "Bob tells me when he can't find one of his toys," she explains. "If he tries to sneak his outside toys into the house, I can always tell by the look on his face. The monkey, stuffed airplane, and plastic newspaper are his indoor toys. If you ask him to bring you the monkey, or any other toy by name, he will. If it's not in his toy basket, he returns with a specific deep moan in a low part of his throat. The placement of his whine and whimper tells me exactly what he is saying. He's totally expressive, more like a teenager than a child." Every other Thursday when Bob goes to the groomers, he always takes his sheepskin teddy bear along for the ride.

If you make a mistake in caring for your pet, try this: apologizing, mirroring, and hearing. Ask him for forgiveness, and mirror back his experience in such a way that he feels "heard." You might say, with your eyes and voice, "I'm so sorry I wasn't here to prepare your dinner on time. I hear that this upset you." Talk to him. Beginning the first day you bring him home, let him become familiar with your voice: its inflection, intent, and tone. He will respond. Let him know that he is validated, respected, and held in high esteem. In return, your animal friend will reward you with an untold depth of love.

Behavioral Clues

If subtle vocal and visual clues do not provide the necessary understanding, observe your pet's behavior. For example, interpreting the actions of Don Quixote, a tomcat, is not difficult, even for the beginner. While his owner is gone for several weeks to visit family overseas, leaving him to be fed by a neighbor, Don methodically pulls sweaters out of drawers and shreds them one by one.

One documentary on house cats concludes that when a cat licks his owner and then grooms himself, it is his way of blending scents and communicating a desire to connect with the caretaker. When a cat grooms his owner, he is expressing the highest form of trust and acceptance. Upon hearing this information, one of my clients was greatly relieved; she had wrongly interpreted her cat's behavior to mean that he wished to rid himself of her scent and maintain a strict separation between them.

Some animal behaviors carry their own undecipherable codes. Instinctual behavior is not based on cruelty any more than it is on kindness. Non-whimsically, non-negotiably, it is based on survival. It has been said by animal-research specialists that the cat's habit of playing with its prey even after it has died is the feline way of calming down after the excitement of the hunt. Perhaps this species-born activity is an exaggerated way of expressing dominance; possibly it is a way of celebrating a victorious hunting session and an innocent reluctance to admit that the party's over. But the most likely interpretation of this behavior is that these actions are defensive and fear-based. The cat wants to make sure his prey is entirely unresponsive before exposing one of his most vulnerable body parts—the face—as he zooms in for the kill. Just watch a cat toying with a spider, much smaller than its size. He will paw and pat and toss it until the threat of its retaliation is a moot point.

Dogs Who Bark Too Much

Dogs bark for a variety of reasons, all of them falling into the category of getting our attention—or our neighbors'—no matter what the underlying motive. Instinctually, barking is a part of canine behavior. Their wolf or coyote ancestors signal to each other through their howling, just as dogs signal to us.

Their yowling can protect us from intruders or imminent danger, based on their steadfast faithfulness to their owners. Recently, front-page headlines in a Santa Rosa, California, newspaper read, "ROHNERT PARK FIRE HEROES—A CAT AND A PUPPY: Two families were saved from a fire early Monday morning by a pair of unlikely heroes: a yellow-eyed cat named Pepper and a frisky puppy called Sammy." When Sammy sensed danger, the young German shepherd–Rottweiler scratched frantically at the door, pacing and whining loudly, awakening his owner and thereby saving their home, a mere ten feet away from the house in flames. Black-coated Pepper, usually sweet-tempered, woke her owners at 3 A.M. by meowing loudly. Opening the door to let her outside, they saw the fire crackling on the exterior of their newly painted home. (History, sometimes in bizarre ways, repeats itself; in 1983, their previous cat's loud, attention-getting whining saved the life of their young son when his electric blanket caught fire.)

Besides barking as a protective mechanism, dogs bark because they are lonely or frustrated. They bark to greet people, cats, and other dogs. They bark if they have not been properly trained. They bark from excitement or restless energy. When injured, they bark in more of a whining manner. If they have been abused, neglected, or otherwise treated badly, they bark out of fear. If treated badly enough, the fear is expressed as aggression, and they bark.

A dog needs to both give and receive companionship. If his owner is home, the dog chained in the yard knows it. Our pack-animal friends are social by nature; even a second dog in the household as a companion for the first can curb a barking problem. Loneliness is often the cause of wandering, digging, and jumping fences. Once we understand a dog's innate nature, we can work with and correct his symptoms of unhappiness. (See also chapter 4, "Behavioral Problems in Pet Owners.")

Dogs are not born afraid or angry. They acquire these qualities through neglect or abuse—sometimes from other animals, but more often from people. And much like people, dogs turn fearful when they are hit, beaten, or slapped. Yes, there are angry dogs, but these are the ones who have been taught to be vicious through improper or inconsistent training or even through roughhousing with children. Most of us think of pit bulls as attack dogs. However, they are actually highly intelligent, keenly loyal, and supremely trainable. People who welcome this breed into their household know firsthand how lovely and kind they are by nature. It is, in fact, improper or deliberate training that renders them vicious.

Dogs are smart; they learn quickly when properly trained. The best training method includes guidelines, rules, and parameters—and consistently sticking to them. Add the ingredient of love, and you have guaranteed success. A good trainer can correct almost any behavioral problem in one session alone.

Here is a rule of thumb about which corrective method to choose for your pet for barking or any other disturbing behavior: Ask yourself how you would like to be treated. Some people consider a shock collar, which administers a small negative-reinforcement shock to the dog's throat with each bark, as a workable solution for a barking problem. Dogs who learn slower than others, of course, must wear the collar for an extended period of time. Another collar option is the battery-operated version that emits a citrus scent, unpleasant to dogs, when they bark. Or there is the more radical option: debarking surgery in which the vocal folds are cut, reducing the dog's voice to a whisper or a hoarsely muted sound. Both the shock collar and the surgery are considered inhumane by animal lovers. Clearly, this book is written to present yet another option, one that is quick-acting, gentle, and extremely effective: the use of flower essences.

Anna Drummond at the Pet Adoption League in Grass Valley, California, says she receives thirty calls a week from pet owners who are abandoning their animals. People claim to have tried everything to keep the pet. A typical scenario is this: puppy gets neglected; puppy starts barking, digging, jumping fences, and running away; and then puppy—now a dog with, literally, life-threatening behavioral problems—gets crazy. In most cases, these problems are completely resolvable. Even strays and dogs who were never trained, Anna reports, will "come around" with lots of love. The final verdict: *There is never a reason to get rid of a dog.* (See chapter 4, "Behavioral Problems in Pet Owners.")

Honey's placement in a new home is but one example. A yellow Lab mix, she was adopted by a couple who wanted an indoor dog to cuddle and spoil.

A previously abandoned and abused dog, Honey is now coming out of her shell of silent neglect, her behavior exemplary in every way. Proper loving care, gentle and consistent discipline, and regular veterinary visits that include worm medicine have transformed this dog into a beloved family member. Sometimes love alone is all it takes to heal an animal.

The following story exemplifies how love, combined with the use of flower essences, can help a dog heal from trauma to a state of receptivity to proper training. In the case of Molly, a five-year-old purebred cocker spaniel, we see an abused, fearful animal transformed into a "perfect little school dog," according to her second owner. Prior to moving to her new home, Molly was raised by a couple who finally divorced, which was the primary reason she was given away. An atmosphere of ambivalence shaped her early environment, from eight weeks to two years old; the woman wanted Molly, the man did not. Upon returning from his night-shift job early each morning and finding Molly on the bed, he would beat her until she awoke and jumped down. As a result, she would nip at him, only making matters worse.

The only day Molly did not bark, reported the new owner, was the day she adopted the gold-coated spaniel. For the next three years, Molly barked loudly and almost incessantly on a daily basis. Men and older boys upset her the most, especially those of large, towering physiques. Barking was exactly the behavior that the new owner, an elementary school teacher, did not want in a dog. Molly's job was to accompany her to school and befriend the children in her classroom. As a breed, cocker spaniels tend to be very affectionate and good with children. A hyperactive and high-strung nature is common among purebreds due to overbreeding. Yet even with an ongoing barking problem, Molly was a well-behaved and loving companion in the classroom, and she never chased the deer on the rural campus.

We started Molly on a single-essence program of Tomato for her fear-based, almost hysterical, barking. The quality and tone of the barking were self-protective, not to guard people or property.

The day after beginning Tomato Essence, Molly had become "more peaceful," the owner reported. "While driving to school, we passed a man jogging alongside the road, and Molly didn't bark as usual. When the kids came to school, she remained quiet—she used to run up and bark at anyone. Now she only barks when someone enters the classroom. Also, she used to walk up to you, turn her back, and sit down. Now she sits and looks at you, making much more direct eye contact."

Within three days, one level of Molly's barking, based on hearing someone approaching the classroom, had completely ceased. Also considerably diminished was the barking initiated by watching someone outside. Behavioral patterns had begun to shift and change.

We had reached a level of receptivity, for the first time, where Molly was responsive to training. In only one phone session with a professional dog trainer, the owner learned a few "tricks" that soon stopped the barking altogether, such as cutting back on Molly's food so that she could be given more treats. The trainer, kind and clear in her assessment of Molly's behavior, said the dog needed to realize that the act of people coming through the doorway is a good experience. So when the children entered the classroom, they would grab a treat stored outside the door and give it to her. In this way, Molly, now trainable, was retrained.

Verbal commands were modified as well. When this previously abused dog had been told "No barking," the command aggravated her problem and created further confusion. According to the trainer, what Molly heard was, "They're after me." Molly was then taught a new word—"Quiet"—to be spoken to her in a gentle and loving manner.

"Listen to your voice," the trainer advised the owner. "Convey the feeling of quietude when speaking to your dog. Words, to an animal, are only a small part of the communication process; the energy behind them is what matters most."

"Molly now gives little verbal greetings," the present owner comments, "but they are happy and not aggressive sounds. A happy greeting sounds different from her previous barking, which conveyed the message, 'I'm not sure about this; maybe you should stand outside the door.'" Excessive barking, for this canine and many others, is a symptom of unhealed emotional pain triggered by abusive treatment. With simple instructions combined with flower essence therapy, Molly is a happy and healthy dog, one who no longer barks incessantly.

Cats: Telltale Tails and Other Behavioral Clues

Cats, although often expressively loving, have earned a reputation for aloof-ness. We might consider their seeming standoffishness as a symptom of a deeper trait: a basic involvement in their own lives, schedules, and needs. For these reasons, cats may seem busy, preoccupied, or even meditative—unless they are sleeping. As one cat enthusiast put it, "Of all the cats I have known, I have never known one with insomnia." And as "many a truth is said in jest," here is a comical explanation of "The Story of Creation" as narrated by a cat:

> On the first day of creation, God created The Cat.
>
> On the second day, God created man to serve The Cat.
>
> On the third day, God created all the animals of the earth to serve as potential food and/or amusement for The Cat.
>
> On the fourth day, God created honest toil so that man could labor for the good of The Cat.
>
> On the fifth day, God created the sparkle ball so that The Cat might or might not play with it.
>
> On the sixth day, God created veterinary science to keep The Cat healthy and the man broke.
>
> On the seventh day, God tried to rest, but he had to scoop out The Litter Box.

For all their reputed inaccessible aloofness as humorously extolled above, cats are a veritable neon display of their innermost selves. From head to tail tip, their body language signals the depth of their thoughts and feel-ings. A cat who looks you in the eyes, lids half-closed, is communicating his comfort with and acceptance of you. When he blinks and turns away, it means you have been acknowledged and then dismissed; he is not inter-ested in further interaction at that time.

The cat's ears, extremely mobile and expressive, communicate many emotional states. When relaxed, they signal happiness, playfulness, calm-ness, or curiosity—unless he is behaving with aggressive confidence. Ears back and lowered are the sign of a cat who feels threatened and is on the defense, the eyes and pupils mere slits, expressing fear or self-protection. Ears alert and upright, combined with eyes wide open and pupils enlarged, means an alert curiosity in a specific object. Ears upright and wide accompanied by a full display of teeth indicates defiance and aggression.

But it is the tail that tells all. Cat tails range in color, width, length, and shape. From three to twenty-eight caudal vertebrae, or tailbones, compose the tail. A cat uses his tail for balance, much like a tightrope walker with an umbrella or balancing pole. This dexterous anatomical wonder allows cats to walk on high, narrow ledges with perfect balance. Pivoting, fast turns, and sudden stops are all maneuvered with this handy instrument. The expression "landing on one's feet" is credited not only to the cat but mainly to the deftness of his tail, which he will instinctively rotate like a propeller in the opposite direction of the intended fall before landing, featherlike, on solid ground. Powerful hind-leg muscles and a flexible spine also make this animal an astounding athlete.

A twitching, upright tail is a welcome-home greeting for you. A slow wag with a slight whipping motion registers annoyance; being otherwise occupied, he prefers solitude and does not wish to be bothered by intruders. A twitch at the very tip of the tail says the cat is ready to pounce on his prey—whether alive or battery-operated. A tail and ears held low accompany the stalking cat who is uncertain of what he is exploring; caution defines this posturing. A fluffed-up tail means the cat feels both threatened and defensive. He is preparing for an attack, if necessary, and making himself look as large and looming as possible. At this time, he may also turn sideways to his aggressor, with arched back and raised fur, again cleverly creating the optical illusion of being much larger than his actual size. Warning: Do not go near an angry cat; he is in "fight or flight" mode and is a veritable tooth-and-claw machine.

In addition to expressing both offensive and defensive maneuvers with his tail, a feline may also express his indecision when petted by his owner. A quick side-to-side flicking indicates both his enjoyment of the attention and an enough-is-enough message, conveyed as diplomatically as he can muster. A tail tipped to one side at the top signifies that the cat is feeling reserved; if completely vertical, he wants to engage in contact. A slightly raised tail also shows interest in communicating or connecting. A tail down, crooked at the tip in a question-mark style, means he is relaxed. Read a cat's tail, and you've got a fascinating autobiography in front of you.

Another seeming feline mystery is their purring sound. Physiologically, when the vocal cords tighten from top to bottom and the cat exhales, the cords are pulled sideways, creating the vibration. Purring expresses contentment and receptivity to attention. Felines purr when nursing or being suckled. Cats also use purring when they have been severely injured, quite possibly as a calming mechanism. A sign of confidence at times, this sound may be an invitation to other household cats that they are comfortably welcomed by the dominant cat.

It is clear that purring is a means for cats to communicate their emotional states. We might compare the cat's purr to the human's smile or even the way people sometimes hum to themselves. Sound is comforting; sometimes we, like the cat, simply enjoy producing it. Over time, we can learn to hear the different messages expressed in our cat's mysterious purr as well as in their meows: hunger, loneliness, or "What's up? I'm bored" dialogue.

Cats, contrary to popular belief, are social animals. They do, however, like to "have their space." All newcomers to the household must understand their role as guests and be accepted on the cats' terms. Cats enjoy companionship, but as they are also highly territorial, a guest may visit only with their express permission. Animal behaviorists concur that, in order for cats to relate readily with people, they need human contact between the ages of two to eight weeks. If little or no connection is made during this stage of imprinting, these felines will be more aloof; they will keep to themselves and not actively seek out human contact, including petting and lap-sitting. Many cats, however, do like to be petted, as it re-creates the sensation of being groomed by their mothers in infancy. Even so, they will let you know when they've had enough and may end a stroking session with a light nipping or by simply walking away.

Moving house, travel, and any number of changes in their living space can be distressing to cats, who are very environment-oriented. Cats do not like being surprised, nor do they appreciate loud noise or other abrupt disturbances. Regularity and sameness are very important to their emotional well-being. For this reason, flower essences are particularly helpful: Pear

Essence, to ease the trauma of change; Corn, for adapting to new situations; Grape, for feeling jealous or neglected in the home; and Raspberry, if it seems that they have been offended or have had their feelings hurt by changes in the owner's life.

Cats relate everything back to themselves. If this dynamic is understood and respected, you will have a contented, well-adjusted cat. If not, soiling, spraying, hissing, and growling are possible resultant behaviors—all expressive of their displeasure.

Dominance, Hierarchy, and Territory

Cats are especially sensitive to feeling replaced. Bringing a new cat or other animal into the household is one of the main problems people report with cats. Usually, one cat will assume the dominant role in the home. If the other cats or pets agree, harmony will pervade. If not, it means trouble. Owners can exacerbate this situation by scolding the dominant cat and rewarding the cat who is bullied. It is actually the dominant cat who needs help, which the owner can provide with support and kindness. Establishing dominance is another form of creating the "space" so important to the feline species.

Cats, as a rule, must never be harshly spoken to; their sensitivity is deeply wounded by stern discipline. Grape Essence is helpful for the dominant cat in this situation, whereas Corn—for adjustment to a new living situation—is often a great help to the newer cat.

Also, one very clever cat-psychology trick for bringing a new cat into the home is to place it in a room with the door closed. This may be called the "entry phase" and will allow the older cat to feel unthreatened by a new cat who has moved into her territory. Hearing the newcomer's meows will awaken her protective, maternal instincts as well as her innate sense of curiosity. It will also give the older cat a sense of being in control with full respect for her seniority and territorialism. No boundaries will be overstepped, and no hierarchy will be trampled.

Butterfly, an eight-month-old kitten, was introduced into the household of Simone, a twelve-year-old house cat. Since both cats had been moved to this new location at the same time, Simone had not had the opportunity to familiarize herself with the new environment. Even so, the owners understood the necessity of respecting her seniority. The entry-phase strategy worked. Almost immediately, with clear lines of dominance established, the two cats bonded easily and got on like old friends. This introduction/bonding process may take several months or even longer, but it may be hastened significantly with the application of flower essences, as illustrated in the following story.

Alexandra, a gray seven-month-old kitten, had bonded beautifully with her new owner—until three-month-old Panda arrived on the scene. Completely unafraid, Alexandra was described as "a people person who loved animals too." She liked playing with the deer outside and rubbing noses with them. Thinking that another kitten in the household would provide companionship for her, the owner found trouble instead. For three weeks, Alexandra growled and hissed at the woman, who easily recognized anger in this new behavior. The interesting point is that Alexandra bonded nicely with Panda; it was to the owner that she exhibited her anger in the form of hissing, stiffening her body, and growling, her teeth exposed.

The owner reported, "I picked up Alexandra yesterday to give her Grape Essence and put it behind her ears. She was growling and didn't want to be held. As soon as I touched her fur with the remedy, she stopped growling. She remained in a stiff posture but became more mellow. She quieted down while I applied the essence. And when I petted her, she stopped growling, though she still looked at me with anger. Then I talked to her and told her, 'I know how angry you are, I know how you feel.' She was looking right at me, then she'd look away. It was really sweet. She's less angry with me now."

The following evening, Alexandra resumed her sleeping position in the bed near her owner's head for the first time in three weeks. The responsive purring also returned, and the growling ceased. "It was breaking my heart," the owner continued, "because she was so mad. I told her that I knew she was angry, that it was OK, and that I was really sorry and really loved her. She heard and acknowledged my words and feelings."

Panda responded immediately to Corn Essence. "He is enjoying being a kitten," the owner said, "following Alexandra around the house, and expressing interest and curiosity in his new surroundings."

Horses

Horses are a highly sensitive and intelligent species. Many horse owners, in fact, say they feel that their animals can read their minds and respond to their cues before any words are spoken. Whether equines are mind-readers or are simply adept at spotting the subtlest body-language clues of their owners and riders; their keen sense of awareness is remarkable. Cantering, trotting, centering, stopping, walking, and reversing on cue are commonly intuited by these graceful twelve-hundred-pound animals.

Equine therapy centers, cognizant of the compassionate nature of these animals, offer programs and workshops for people suffering from emotional and physical problems. Horses seems to intuit the special needs of humans; they work well with people suffering from paralysis, cerebral palsy, autism, and brain injury.

It is this acuity that allows a horse to be exceptionally responsive to subtle remedies such as flower essences. Little Guy, a young Arabian stallion, had weathered an unusually wet winter that had created lush, grassy fields for the herd. The horses were thriving on the greenery as well as enjoying the absence of ticks, which had been killed off by the uncommon moisture. This herd was "feeling its oats" and had been well fattened by the rich green diet.

Since the heavy rains and slick fields had prevented the horses from being ridden as usual, their owner decided one morning to groom them one by one, bringing them in and tying them to a hitching post. Arabians tend to have an excitable nature, and Little Guy was no exception. When his turn came, he began galloping in place, disturbed by the break in routine and temporary separation from his family. The owner placed two drops of Pear on her fingers and rubbed them into Little Guy's nostrils. Within three minutes, he had calmed down completely. Had the essence not been applied, it is unlikely that anything done in this situation would have restored his equilibrium.

Equine sensitivity readily lends itself to flower essence therapy, as recounted in the following story. A three-year-old Arabian stallion who had been boarded at a cattle ranch had become overexcited by all the commotion of the roundup. Later that morning, his owner led him to a stall in the barn to calm him down. Stallions are territorial, and hearing the confused commotion, he began pacing and calling nervously. Just ten minutes after applying Pear to his nostrils, an astonished and grateful owner found him napping in his stall. Without the essence, there would have been no calming him.

Ferrets

Ferrets are members of the *mustela furo* family, *furo* meaning "little thief." They are closely related to otters, skunks, minks, weasels, polecats, and badgers. Two thousand years of domestication have tamed this little creature, save for the wild, endangered black-footed ferret of North America. A tamed ferret can no longer survive in the wild if he is let loose; he might kill a mouse but would no longer possess the instinct to eat it. In the United States, Hawaii and California still consider the ferret to be wild; owning them in these states is illegal.

Ferrets love to play; their antics will leave you in stitches. The more excited they become, the less coordinated are their theatrics. As ferrets in the wild will hunt prey twice their size, such as rabbits, you may see them dragging your shoe off to their lair. Their natural memory capabilities allow them to remember exactly where they have hidden your possessions, much like a squirrel burying his winter stash of acorns.

Their forms of play mimic their activities in nature: hunting, nurturing, foraging, and hoarding. One eight-year-old ferret owner describes his pet as follows: "He does backflips off my bed and stuff. When he really gets going, he will accidentally do a flip and then slam into the furniture. He's really smart. He always explores and figures stuff out. He loves to play tug-of-war." And although ferrets will retain their playfulness throughout their lives, the younger ones are fidgety whereas the older ones become more cuddly.

As a species, ferrets are wound up and intensely active. Houdini, a young ferret described by his owner as "a little guy who bounces off the walls," is another example of Lettuce Essence's gentle approach. After a few days with Lettuce Essence added to his water bottle, the owner reported that he no longer nips and is not quite as rambunctious—though he remains extremely playful and fun to watch.

Rabbits

Over forty rabbit breeds exist in the United States. Rabbits are bright, inquisitive, playful, and easy to care for. But as baby rabbits tend to be adorably cuddly, impulse buying without proper education about their care is the main cause of rabbits ending up homeless in shelters and rescue facilities. As a species, their emotional states and needs differ somewhat from larger animals such as horses, cats, and dogs. Like other small household pets, they more often play the role of prey than predator in the wild, and they naturally bring this instinctual memory into domesticated existence. Fear of loud noises or large objects, including people; loneliness from being left alone or not having other rabbits' companionship; and disorientation with relocation or changes in their environment are commonly treated in this species by Tomato, Grape, and Pear Essences, respectively.

Rabbits respond beautifully to flower essences. Their gentle nature suggests a receptivity to the more sensitive methods of treatment. One little girl, the owner of a family of rabbits whose cage leans against her house, described a tragic occurrence for her rabbit family. Shortly after the mother had given birth to five babies, a rattlesnake entered the cage, biting all but one of the newborns, Lilly, and the father, Freckles. In trying to protect her young, the mother was also attacked; she passed away that evening. Since that time, Lilly would not allow her young owner to pick her up for cuddling. The young girl suspected Lilly's reason: the last thing she saw the girl do with her mother was pick her up and remove her from the cage. Lilly never saw her mother again.

Freckles, too, had behaved listlessly since all in his family but Lilly had died. His owner noticed that he now grooms Lilly, a new behavior since his partner passed away. "Freckles became both the mom and dad when she died," she noticed. "He really loved the babies. He used to nudge them, train them to walk, and wrestle gently with them." His owner commented that Freckles had remained more withdrawn since the babies died. With only two rabbits left in an outdoor cage, one will stand guard while the other takes a nap. Whether this behavior is instinctual or familial remains to be seen.

The young girl reported an immediate change in Lilly's behavior when Orange Essence was added to her morning water: "Lilly hopped right up to me when I gave them their water with the essence in it. She jumped right in the cage and started drinking for a long time, and this is not normal for her. Both she and Freckles are not so scared and nervous-looking anymore." And although Tomato Essence—for the fear and terror of the rattlesnake entering their cage—would be a reasonable choice in this situation, the predominant need for both rabbits was to address their grieving from the loss of their family members, indicating Orange Essence.

Birds

Birds are amazing companions for people of all ages. Elderly people who are hospitalized or who are living in nursing homes, according to studies by the University of Nebraska Medical Center, report that the company of pet birds and other animals reduces the sense of loneliness, helplessness, and boredom, not to mention the depression experienced in long-term care institutions.

One owner of an outdoor aviary of forty birds, mostly parakeets and cockatiels, explains how loving and responsive they are. After a time, she began to notice that they would let her know what they wanted by singing, whistling, or making direct one-on-one contact. Interpreting their body language, she observed that they would move their heads in one direction or another, depending on what they wished her to do. They recognized and responded to their own names. Birds love being quietly sung to and will respond with their own voices. Some of the males would sing back to the owner, and thus she would know if they wanted company or whether being able to see her at some distance away in the garden sufficed.

At certain times of the day, the birds would intuit her visit and begin singing to her. One bird even learned to whistle a particular song she was accustomed to singing. They would express their territorial instincts by perching on her shoulders, one bird on each side. In fact, they responded to one-on-one behavior, letting down their guard when they could have her individual attention.

Lovebirds—so named because they attach themselves to one partner—bond very strongly with each other, regardless of gender. They will connect with a family or another bird and remain lifetime partners, much like best friends. Pairing off and huddling together on a perch are common behaviors for them. If these social little parrots do not have a mate, they will form an enduring bond with a human friend. Lovebirds are flock animals; for their well-being, they need company while playing and eating.

When a "spouse" dies, their sense of loss is immense and deeply disturbing, as illustrated in the following story. Katrina, a two-year-old peach-faced lovebird, had lost her mate. Katrina never allowed anyone to touch her, remaining constantly skittish. Typically, when one partner dies, the remaining lovebird will pine away. When a new partner was introduced into her cage, she remained unconnected and was unable to bond with him. Even in a relatively small cage, she kept her distance and continued to behave in a withdrawn manner.

After one day with Orange Essence, for grief, added to her drinking water, she warmed to her new partner. Reported her twelve-year-old owner, "I think the Orange Essence is doing really well for Katrina, because when the other bird is in a snuggly mood, he makes this funny sound with his beak and does all these really weird dancing things, and I saw them doing this together on a stick. I never saw them doing this together before. So that's really amazing. She seems much happier and more excited."

Wild birds also respond wonderfully to flower essences—Pear in particular. One woman who lives in the countryside reports that hummingbirds routinely fly into her house through an open door and then repeatedly slam against a closed window in an attempt to escape. Trapping them in a scarf, she will apply a few drops of Pear to their beaks and then watch them fly off, apparently free from injury. With the shock of physical harm lessened or removed and their life force restored, the birds easily regain flight.

Anthropomorphism Reversed

Animals, instinctively intuitive, have no trouble reading *us*. Lion tamers can command fear in the animals they train with no more gesturing than striding into a cage. Birds flocked and perched freely upon the shoulders of

St. Francis of Assisi. Animals both read and respond to inner consciousness, not outward appearance. Those who have mastered the quality of *ahimsa*— a Sanskrit word meaning harmlessness, and also the philosophy popularized by Mahatma Gandhi—find that even ferocious, untamed animals become gentle in their presence. How transparently readable we are to them!

Domestic and wild animals, living on a level of awareness of the third *kosha* mentioned in chapter 1, are "personalities in process." All anthropomorphism aside, animals who spend time in the company of humans actually do begin to imitate their behaviors—to take on likes and dislikes, to express preferences. A dog may show pride in his ability to do good deeds. A cat, highly territorial by nature, may turn resentful if another pet is brought into the household. Animals, endowed with richly emotional natures, are capable of delight, enjoyment, curiosity, and a sense of adventure as their awareness expands.

Just as people of different nationalities possess general characteristics, so different animals possess traits particular to their species. "Monkey see, monkey do" is an apt generalization of primates, who delight in imitating whatever they see. The fox is stereotyped for his slyness, cunning, and expertise in thievery, especially where chickens are concerned. "Playing possum," too, is an accurate description for the mammal who feigns a deathlike sleep as a survival skill to confound his predators. To be lion-hearted is the embodiment of bravery, and the lion kills only when hungry and not out of mere viciousness or for the sake of the hunt. The house cat is hygienic and basically aloof, tending to its own needs. The horse is quick and of high intelligence. The gentle dove has become an archetypal symbol for peace and meekness.

Consider, then, this reversal of *anthropomorphism*, a term that means attributing human motivations, characteristics, or behaviors to animals. If animals can behave like people, the reverse is also true. People may express animal-like qualities—some positive and innocent, some replete with guile. We see the cunning businessman who, fox-like, financially secures a business deal at the expense of his clients. The "Simon says" individual, lacking an integrity of his own and merely imitating through fashions or fads, mimics the monkey.

Human company hastens the evolution of animals. In fact, we may distinguish domesticated animals from those in the wild on this one point alone: pets develop relationships with people, whereas wild animals, in general, do not. Out of this connection is born the dearest possible bond: friendship. Referring back to our new definition of a pet—"an animal whom we domesticate in exchange for providing the highest possible quality of care"—this means tending to them *with the highest possible awareness on our part.* With loving sensitivity, we can help our pets to deepen their natural intuition and sharpen their attention, which in turn supports their physical health. Among the more refined tools at our disposal for this purpose are flower essences. Love, too, can transport us into their world.

4

BEHAVIORAL PROBLEMS
IN PET OWNERS

Properly trained, a man can be dog's best friend.
Corey Ford

I recently interviewed Sonya Fitzpatrick, an internationally acclaimed animal communicator and author of *What the Animals Tell Me*. "I often find when people come to me to solve a problem," she related, "it isn't people with an animal problem. It's the other way around, I tell you, in nine out of ten cases. It's an animal with an owner problem."

When we accept that we, the owners, are often contributors to our pets' problems, we can begin to repair these imbalances at their primary source: possibly, us. And just as flower essences do not replace proper veterinary care, they also do not replace proper attention from the owner. Thus, the seemingly unrelated subtopics in this chapter all have one thing in common: each issue, if not health-related, will provide anywhere from a subtle clue to an outright demand from the animal who is expressing in no uncertain terms that something in his world is amiss.

The purpose of this chapter is to help us become more aware as pet owners through realistically assessing our needs as well as those of our pets. Once we understand that, by far, most of the problems people encounter with their pets are not temperamental but behavioral in nature, we can then correct these issues. This means that the problems lie, not in the individual personalities of the animals but in their actions that either upset our peace of mind or destroy our home and property, or both.

Much like animals with their species, breed, and genetic codes, the behavior of human beings is also somewhat dictated by instinctual and sociobiological factors. Rather than breeds, however, we use the terms *cultures* or *nationalities*. And just as individuals have personalities, so do large groups of people. Consider, for example, the basic personality of the American culture, which is hallmarked by its humanitarian spirit, go-getter attitude, quick-thinking nature, and great kindliness. Americans make fine pet owners based on these qualities.

At the same time, a certain fickleness and lack of commitment pervade the basic American makeup, reflected in its marriage statistics. America, with half its marriages legally terminated, carries the highest divorce rate of any country in the world. An expressed lack of enduring commitment is a trait to be reckoned with where pet adoption is being considered.

In essence, there are basically two kinds of people who own animals: those who would do anything for them, who love them as respected family members, whose lives are changed through the sharing of loving companionship with animals; and those who, respectively, won't, don't, and aren't. Just as having children does not necessarily make one a good parent, likewise owning pets may not create a genuine pet owner. Sonya Fitzpatrick also shared that "real animal lovers work with their pets. You usually find that they don't have a lot of problems with them."

In the introduction, I talked about redefining the word *pet*. It cannot be overemphasized that the responsibility of claiming a pet is lifelong. Indeed, the kitty or puppy for purchase outside the supermarket is cute and cuddly and supremely salable. But what happens when the kitty claws the curtains and couch or the puppy barks morning and night? Caring for a pet means a lifetime commitment—their lifetime. At this juncture, it is helpful for potential pet owners to assess their own needs, capabilities, and circumstances.

Why People Give Their Pets Away

To summarize exactly why people relinquish their animals, the problem is simply a lack of awareness. People are often not aware of what is involved in pet care. Pet owners, in essence, are usually not properly trained or educated beforehand. In turn, many people do not train their pets and yet expect them to be perfect. Dogs, for example, will naturally jump up on people unless they are consistently trained not to do so. A lack of awareness leads to disastrous situations, and these unfortunate circumstances are completely avoidable.

It is easy to romanticize the concept of having a pet; the reality, however, is another story altogether. Imagine a walk in the woods with your trusty canine companion. The sun sparkles on the leaves, the endorphins pump gently through your body. Then, imagine having to walk the dog every day. The days turn to weeks; the weeks become tiresome years. Other chores pile up interminably: the laundry, the phone calls for the PTA, the visits with relatives. How long until this beautiful dog becomes a burden?

Most pets who are abandoned or given away are between five months to three years of age; most have lived with their present guardian for less than a year. The highest number relinquished are obtained through friends. Almost half of these animals (specifically cats and dogs) are not neutered and have never received veterinary care.

According to the National Council on Pet Population Study and Policy, these are the top ten reasons people give their pets away:

1. The family is moving to a new home.
2. The landlord does not allow pets.
3. There are too many animals in the home.
4. The cost of maintaining the pet is too high.
5. The pet owner is having personal problems.
6. The facilities are inadequate.
7. The home cannot accommodate litter mates.
8. For dogs: There is not enough time to care for the pet. For cats: Allergies in the family require the pet to leave.
9. For dogs: Pet illness is a key factor. For cats: House soiling is a major problem.
10. For dogs: Biting is a serious problem. For cats: Incompatibility with other household pets warrants the animal being relocated.

Our Commitment

Once removed from their natural habitats, animals are not self-supporting. Telling the cat to go out and get a job doesn't work. It is our job, and our privilege, to meet their needs on every level. This translates as food, shelter, healthcare, companionship, and above all, love. At the same time, when we remove animals from their natural habitats and bring them into our home and property, their natural behaviors may no longer be acceptable. The ferret's sharp-toothed nipping, for example, is not pleasant and may become annoying over time. The colt's bucking and rearing is outright dangerous. Animals need to adjust to our ways, and we to theirs, by finding a happy medium that creates a comfortable living situation for both.

People love their pets. Yet abuse happens. Pets can be frustrating for people who do not have the time, the funds, or the emotional ability to blend their lives with their pets'. Without the necessary willingness, receptivity, and flexibility on the owner's part, pets can be burdensome. "If my cat doesn't stop spraying in the house," reported one pet owner of her eleven-year-old house companion, "he'll have to go to the pound." Spraying, noise, aggression, and other unpleasant or inconvenient behaviors are several significant reasons that people send their pets to animal shelters. From there they may be placed in other homes, but all too often they are simply put to death.

Euthanasia is the sad fate for many hundreds of thousands of animals whose behavior is upsetting to humans. Quite often, unwanted behaviors can be traced back to poor training at best and outright abuse at worst. Or the owner may inadvertently be contributing to the pet's problem, sometimes merely through lack of education or information. Animals have an instinctual ability to intuit their owner's emotional states. A troubled owner is often mirrored in a troubled pet (see chapter 6).

The sorry statistics for dogs and cats who are euthanized each year are staggering. And we are responsible. For example, the redemption rate for cats—meaning that someone comes to the pound to reclaim them—is 2 percent. More and more no-kill shelters are springing up across the country, where animals are not put to sleep unless they are severely ill or aggressive. Even elderly animals can be placed in homes, and dogs are groomed and trained before being relocated with new families. Great efforts are being made through the media to encourage people to find their animal companions at shelters and pounds.

With growing frequency, flower essences are being recognized as a viable and often life-saving alternative to pet abandonment. Essence therapy can help sensitize owners to their pet's needs. Flower essences treat the cause of a problem, not its effects. If the cause resides in the pet owners' care of the animal, it is they we must treat with flower essences and counseling.

Selecting Your Pet

Some pet authorities suggest taking as much time and energy to select a pet as you would to invest in a new car. I would like to propose that you give this decision as much consideration as bringing a child into your life. Here are some points for honest self-assessment about welcoming an animal into your household or property. Are you willing to

- Clean the cage, stall, yard, bedding, or litter as often as needed for the animal's comfort and hygiene?
- Clean after he messes up where he is not supposed to?
- Give your pet special care when he is ill or older, i.e., medications or special treatments?
- Risk the soiling or shredding of your belongings, including indoor and outdoor plants or trees?
- Take the time for proper litter/yard training?
- Rearrange your home and/or land to make them pet-proof, i.e., fine china stored safely out of reach, or a sturdy fenced area provided in the yard?
- Adjust your work, social life, vacation time, and basic routine to include your pet's needs?
- Board your pet or have him house-sat or fed and given companionship while you are gone on vacation or business trips so that his needs are consistently met during your absence?
- Never leave your pet alone in a vehicle while you are out running errands?
- Spend the necessary fees, possibly expensive at times, for proper veterinary care?
- Find time in your schedule around other activities for yourself and your family to arrange vet visits, obedience training sessions, or whatever else is needed for your pet?
- Spend the necessary amount for a nourishing diet and any additional supplements?
- Take time to prepare meals for your pet, even if you have other family members, as this responsibility often rests with the adult or, especially, with children in the household?

- Have your pet spayed or neutered to avoid contributing to a critical overpopulation problem?
- Educate yourself on vaccinations or viable replacements and follow the program?
- Supply proper grooming tools as well as toys for entertainment and exercise?
- Walk your dog, play with your cat, ride your horse; in other words, spend active, quality time with your pet?

In addition, consider your answers to the following questions:

- What is your reason for wanting a pet: companionship, a friend for your children, etc.?
- Is your living space of adequate size for your pet? Does it pose any dangers or hazards?
- Will neighbors be disturbed and possibly complain?
- How much time will the animal have to spend alone each day, week, and month?
- Does the animal you are considering match your special needs and temperament?
- Are you able to work with the frustrations and stress of your own life without venting these tensions on your pet?
- What are his particular breed or species needs for companionship with people or other pets?
- How much special care and companionship does the animal require before it reaches maturity?
- Recognizing that a baby animal is cute, are you willing to care for him as a much heavier and larger pet?
- Are you properly educated about the particular breed or species of animal you are bringing into your home? What are his particular physical and emotional needs? Behaviors? Grooming habits?
- If children live in the home with you, are they allergic to this kind of animal? Do they understand how to care for the pet? If not, will they be trained and educated as well?

- Are you willing to care for the pet if and when your children lose interest once the novelty of a pet has worn thin—usually in about one week?
- How mobile is your lifestyle? Are you able to provide a stable, routine environment for your pet whether you are present or absent?

Loneliness is a serious condition for people and pets alike. If our motive in adopting a pet is to remedy our own sense of lack, we need to be certain that the favor is reciprocated. Your animal's health can be seriously affected by recurring states of abandonment, rejection, depression, stress, anxiety, anger, or replacement by another pet.

Does your work require regular business trips such that pets have to deal with your absence from home on a recurring basis? If so, they need special care from loving sitters while you are away to minimize the household's changing climate. One cat enthusiast and author suggests that when we leave home for an extended period of time, our pets worry—and justifiably so. Their projected assumption is that you have gone out hunting and have been eaten by a predator.

Some important allowances in the home will need to be made to accommodate your pet. Depending on the breed you have chosen, good household practices include allowing your pet safe access to the outdoors balanced with an indoor environment as free of toxins as possible: chemical-free carpeting, lead-free paint, and nontoxic household cleansing agents. Such commonly used chemicals, ingested as he grooms himself, are devastating to your pet's health.

In addition, animals should never, ever, be struck. And although this point may seem so obvious that it ought not even be mentioned—especially to the audience of a book of this nature—many of my animal clients have been beaten or otherwise abused by previous owners. Serious damage can be done to them physically and emotionally, inhibiting their ability to form trusting bonds with people.

Some owners who come to my office for consultation explain that they want their pets to behave in a way that is contrary to the animal's breed, species, personality, or age. This situation usually indicates a mismatch of the pet's personality with that of the owner. Ask yourself before acquiring a pet if you are prepared to take on the animal's particular behaviors. An infinitely adventurous, finely wired creature such as an Abyssinian cat may be entertaining for a while, but are you ready for year after year of their ever-new inquisitiveness and inherent desire to explore the icebox, your new shoes, and the water dripping in the kitchen sink? For instance, a high-strung chihuahua is best matched with a high-energy owner. An older lapcat can be the perfect companion for a sedentary owner. It is important to add here that flower essences will not alter behavior in ways foreign to the animal's true nature. Essences do not control or manipulate; rather, they allow the animal's unique individuality to come forth in its most positive expression.

"The Litter-Box Blues"

Perhaps the greatest problem of cat owners is related to the litter box. At least 10 percent of cats, at some time in their lives, will soil, or defecate outside the litter box. Understanding the reasons why a cat soils inside the home, ruling out health problems assessed by a qualified veterinarian and the condition of the box and litter, is a straightforward case of analyzing the animal's motives. More often than not, he is expressing severe upset with the behavior of his owner.

Kittens are trained by their natural mothers at three to four weeks of age to either use the box or, if outdoors, to find a patch of land with soft dirt or sand. Once trained, cats retain this knowledge and should not need to be retrained. Instinct teaches cats to cover their scent in order to avoid alerting predators to their presence. Litter-box problems—understandably considered by cat owners as their primary misbehavior—are completely correctable.

Ruling out physical problems such as kidney or bladder weakness, arthritis (which makes it difficult for older cats to reach the box), wrong diet, or a need for neutering, cats can make no statement stronger than soiling the very territory over which they reign. Keeping the litter box spotlessly clean is essential. Some cats act as though they couldn't care less about a dirty box; others get absolutely irate and cannot bear the mess. These are the felines who would much prefer a clean spot of carpet or bedding; they don't seem to mind excreting elsewhere, as long as it's not in an unclean litter box!

Another reason worth investigating is that your cat may not like the particular brand of litter. One study reports that cats prefer sandy-type litters rather than larger pellet-shaped brands. Caution in selecting a product free of drying agents, colors, and deodorizers will save your cat from these toxic substances. Current studies link the clumping clay litters to many serious health problems, such as intestinal disorders, respiratory illnesses, and poorly functioning immune systems. Some excellent organic clumping wheat and corn kernel litters—fresh-scented, dust-free, and completely nontoxic—are now available. Also, cats seem to opt for the open rather than closed box style. Sometimes merely moving the litter box to the cat's preferred location will resolve the problem.

Please note that spraying is a somewhat different issue, although the motives behind the two behaviors may overlap. Marking, as it is also called, is a cat's way of communicating, often in response to strange odors or new people in the house. It is his way of saying, "You can't come in." As a sign of territorialism, he may mark the drapes or the door if he sees another cat through the window.

New carpet or vinyl flooring introduces foreign odors into the cat's territory. Cats operate more through their sense of smell than vision. They are generally not happy with olfactory changes different from the previous familiar scent, and they tend to dislike chemical odors. Instinct may drive them to replace it with their own scent through marking.

Spraying is typically a problem for unneutered males or cats who, feeling instinctively threatened or driven to establish dominance, need to mark their territory. Cats who are neutered when they are older are typically the ones who continue spraying. Especially if the cat is spraying on or near a door or doorway, he may be marking his territory. And here is where training complemented with flower essences becomes an integral part of the solution.

In any case, it is important to thoroughly clean the soiled area with an organic enzymatic cleanser as quickly as possible. An ammonia-based product will only exacerbate the problem, as cat urine contains this chemical. And their grooming of ammonia and other chemical toxins from their paws and coats is extremely harmful to them. Thoroughly cleaning the area will eliminate odors and remove the olfactory invitation for the cat to repeat the action.

Felines are supremely hygienic by nature. A problem with eliminating outside the litter box is an unequivocal demand for attention to issues that cats find deeply disturbing. They deliberately employ this maneuver as a sign of their outrage with our behavior, usually for some way that we have been insensitive to their needs. In fact, the location where cats soil and spray is the most significant clue as to why they are doing it. Punishment for this behavior is one of the worst things an owner can do to the feline species. Especially if reprimanded more than three to five seconds after the soiling occurs—as it is nearly impossible to catch them in the act—cats cannot associate their behavior with the punishment. Instead, such actions may backfire and the cat may begin to fear both the owner and the environment.

With a little of our own detective work—analyzing what changes occurred in the cat's life at the time the problem began—we quickly learn that there is no such thing as an "accident." Litter-box problems are not arbitrary; there is always a reason. The root cause can easily be traced back to something happening in the home. One woman reported that her sweet-tempered nine-year-old house cat began defecating on the bathroom mat—on the very spot where she would step when exiting the shower—exactly at the same time that she began a new relationship. How symbolic a gesture! The cat seemed to know her most vulnerable spot, all the better to get his message across.

We may accurately generalize that litter-box problems indicate an unacceptable behavior by the cat's owner. One man, himself fastidiously tidy, recently reported a serious problem with Junior, a two-year-old neutered house cat. Junior had begun urinating everywhere in the house but on the bed. Junior's new behavior contrasted strongly with his initial integration into his new home as a loving, affectionate cat, delighted with his new circumstances and attentive owner.

At first, Junior urinated only on the doorway; then, on the walls and carpets in every room. When questioned, the owner explained that nothing had changed in his life at the time the rampage began. The man had started a new relationship a few months ago at about the same time he brought Junior into his home. At least superficially, this did not seem to follow the standard pattern of a cat feeling replaced or displaced.

And yet as the love relationship progressed, the owner began to focus more time and energy on his new partner than on Junior, who, by the way, was fondly accepting of the woman. A cat does not so much mind his owner extending love to other animals or people; what irks him to the point of soiling is feeling replaced.

Junior's owner had even begun affectionately referring to his girlfriend as "Kitty Number One"; the cat was then relegated to the role of "Kitty Number Two." Apparently, this conveyed a clear message to Junior that he had been bumped. In addition, the man noted that Junior's play had grown increasingly more aggressive; he used his claws and teeth in a vicious rather than fun-loving manner.

I suggested to the owner that he give Grape Essence to Junior; that he apologize and explain to him that he was in no way being replaced; and, through his eyes, voice, and mental pictures, that he communicate to his feline friend that he was still "Number One" in the owner's heart. Flower essences, combined with behavioral changes on the part of the pet owner, are a veritable remedy for success. (Whereas Grape and Raspberry are the most commonly used essences for litter-box problems—both addressing hurt feelings and highly emotional issues, to which cats as a species are prone—other essences may come into play from time to time.) The owner reported by phone, "Junior's really turned the corner. He's happier, more secure again, and just a jovial little fella."

To summarize, here is a checklist of questions to ask yourself if you get a case of "the litter-box blues."

1. Have you ruled out physical causes for your cat's behavior?
2. If not, has he been diagnosed and treated by a veterinarian?
3. Is the litter box kept clean enough to invite your cat to use it?
4. Does he appear to like the brand of litter, expressed through burying his waste?
5. Is the litter box easily accessible?

6. What changes occurred in your household at the time the problem began?
7. Is there a new pet or partner in the home?
8. Are there stray animals within the property boundaries that he considers his territory?
9. Are people leaving or arriving at this location?
10. Have you or other household members recently left on a trip?
11. If so, did the care given to your cat in your absence meet his needs for food, grooming, play, and most of all, companionship?
12. If you were viewing the situation from your cat's perspective, what changes would you perceive as upsetting to him?

Cats Who Claw

Undesirable behavior in cats such as scratching furniture is a symptom of one of two problems, or sometimes both: improper training, or being confined to a domesticated environment that does not allow proper outlets for their energy. Felines must have exercise; cats need to play. Many of their games, in fact, mimic their instinctual activities in the wild: the stalk-and-pounce or chase-and-catch routines simulating normal hunting maneuvers. Their favorite toys will often be those that mimic the movement of smaller prey animals with feathers or tail-like appendages. Sometimes cats scratch out of boredom; mostly, they like to scratch, stretch, climb, and play to utilize their territory. A cat in the outdoors is a natural roamer; if he is restricted indoors, he may scratch furniture, doors, walls, draperies—and your legs.

The obvious workable solution to scratching is a good scratching post—one that is sturdy enough to resist being knocked over and high enough for a good, lengthy hind-leg stretch. With the decorative and cleverly designed assortment of trees, penthouses, and clubhouses now available, cat furniture can be an elegant addition to the home decor. Kitty heaven is filled with this kind of feline furniture!

If cats aggressively scratch people, there may be another reason for their clawing. They may be either highly unsocialized and primarily feral or expressing serious emotional or medical problems. In these cases, it is important to determine the cause of the problem so that proper treatment may then be administered. A naturally aggressive, destructive domesticated cat is a rare animal.

Clearly the most radical approach to a cat's tendency to scratch is declawing. Onychectomy, as it is called, is a controversial surgical procedure. It involves an irreversible amputation of the cat's claw and most or all of the last bone in the toe. Declawing is illegal in the United Kingdom. Removal of the cat's singular form of instinctive protection, barring his teeth as a last resort, can be summed up in one word: barbaric. One cat authority likens the process to amputating a person's fingertips.

Cats who have been declawed tend to die younger as well as to exhibit troubled behaviors such as extreme fright and paranoia. Infection from the surgery itself is common. In addition, declawing can promote litter-box problems. Being unable to scoop litter without pain, it is only natural that they would soil in areas where they do not have to bury their waste. One cat expert explains, quite simply, "Declawing bunches up their bodies." Cats use their claws to stretch the muscles in their bodies by way of grabbing onto a tree or post as a form of exercise. Uninformed people tend to assume that, since some veterinarians promote this procedure, it can't be all bad, especially with the rationalization that the hind-leg claws are left intact.

If declawing is used as an attempt to cure a cat's aggressive behavior, the owner should be forewarned that the animal may simply resort to a backup weapon: his teeth. It cannot be stressed strongly enough that treating the cause of the problem with a loving flower essence program can alleviate the need for such drastic and damaging measures.

Often if not always, simply retraining a cat who claws furniture or curtains is all that is necessary. When the cat tears into the couch or draperies, some people find that shaking an empty soda can with a few coins in the bottom affords excellent results. Most successful of all, and least traumatic, is double-sided masking tape or its pet-store equivalent applied to the furniture that is off limits to the cat. This method is a brilliant psychological ploy; cats as a species shun the indignity of walking on sticky surfaces. (In fact, one veteran hunter on safari marked his campsite boundaries with flypaper to prevent any unwanted intrusions from wild tigers.) Scratching posts, readily available and in plain view, offer the cat an acceptable alternative.

Sometimes cats like to be playful and "just plain ornery." Even so, they are keenly intelligent and trainable. Consistent training and designated scratching areas, combined with the use of flower essences, ensure a successful end to the ruining of household property. Avocado Essence is an excellent choice for training your cat or other pet, as it promotes alert attention to the subject at hand. Pineapple can boost his sense of achievement, and Fig may help him to develop a healthy sense of parameters in which to learn new behaviors. Praise and rewards make the discipline process agreeable as well as acceptable to your cat.

Dogs on Drugs

Wrong behaviors warrant correction—for both the comfort of the owner and the happiness of the pet. Dr. John Heinerman, veterinarian and author of *Natural Pet Cures*, offers this insightful parallel between inappropriate, aggressive animal and human behavior. Consider the legal consequences if a person were to engage in any of the following activities that are typically ascribed to canines. Such conduct would warrant anything from a ticket to a jail term.

Jump on another person	**Assault**
Bite or scratch someone else without provocation	**Mayhem**
Chase or attack another person for no reason	**Aggravated assault**
Make excessive noise in the household or neighborhood	**Disorderly conduct**
Use someone's front lawn or public sidewalk as a toilet	**Plain lewdness**
Dig a hole in the neighbor's backyard	**Criminal mischief**
Trespass on private property without permission	**Trespassing!**

Unruly behavior can be life-threatening for a dog, especially with complaints from the neighbors. Only last year, the first FDA-approved psychotropic drug specifically for animals appeared on the market. One pharmaceutical company that produces this pet anti-anxiety drug expects annual sales to reach $25 million.

Both humans and animals alike may experience separation anxiety. Frankly, being left alone is depressing. Dogs, who are people-oriented by nature, can now be given a chemical tranquilizer or antidepressant to prevent them from tearing up a house or exhibiting other unwanted behaviors when left alone for long periods of time.

Being pack animals, social ostracizing is a form of death sentence to dogs, according to Dr. Stephen Sundlof, head of the FDA's center for veterinary medicine. Following their instincts, dogs need to bond with other dogs or human families for their health and well-being. Of the 54 million dogs in this country, 10 percent exhibit behavioral problems as a result of being left alone too often in homes or yards. And 40 percent of this group are critically in need of help. Yes, drugs are an option, and greatly preferred over euthanasia. Yet, another choice is available in addition to medicating your animal. Flower essences treat both the pet and the owner by getting to the root of the problem: the pet's loneliness and the owner's inadvertent contribution to leaving him alone at home.

I recently consulted with the owner of Bonnet, a basset hound–beagle mix, who reported a problem with moping and sadness. Bonnet is fine when people are present and, in fact, has such a sweet disposition that neighbors have offered to take care of her when the owner is gone. In her six and a half years, Bonnet is now on her fourth owner. She spends a great deal of time alone in the house, as her owner works and is routinely gone overnight on business trips. When we understand that dogs are a people-oriented species, this fact sheds light on the true cause of the problem: neglect. We might love our pet to be at home to greet us and to fill parts of our days with genuine companionship, but the animal's situation needs to be accounted for as well. This dynamic illustrates a definite need for Grape Essence for the owner—for abandoning a pet without understanding how the animal's life is affected.

Pets and Children

Dogs generally love children. So do birds, rabbits, cats, and horses. If behavioral problems arise in dogs, for example, it is wise to monitor the behavior of the children with the dogs. Dogs are driven to bite or scratch when they are pulled, tugged, or hugged too hard. The bottom line is that people with a vicious animal have done something to make him that way, unless a previous owner is at fault.

Families that house dogs and children together will find a wonderful opportunity to encourage responsibility and kindness in their kids, as the following story conveys. When one child smacked the household dog with a newspaper, the mother, whose motive was to teach her son compassion, asked him how he would feel if someone hit him. This parent successfully conveyed to her child the message of the Golden Rule: Do unto your pets as you would have them do unto you.

Another theory is that children are cruel to animals because they receive cruelty from their role models. Children will kick a dog because they have been kicked. They will punch an animal because they themselves have been abused. And, sadly, children who are afraid to talk about the abuse they receive from their parents will talk openly about how daddy is abusing the dog.

Training's the Name of the Game

Nearly everyone who has attended a dog-training session warranted by a problem with a household dog will admit that the difficulty lies with the owner and not with the dog. The Alpha-dog theory, based on dogs and wolves sharing the same genetic makeup, states that the dog, like his wolf ancestor, looks up to his owner as the head dog of the social pack. Whereas it is not necessary to use the wolf's tactics of growls and bared teeth to force a dog into submission, the canine will defer to and respect your role as a consistent, strong, and fair leader. Harmony prevails in the pack or human family when the owner, as the "alpha animal," makes the rules and enforces them.

Trainers emphasize that it is important to be firm and to mean what you say, especially with the more stubborn breeds. Train a dog not to jump on people, and he will respond, if his response to your commands is rewarded with praise and affection. Your dog will respect your role as "leader of the pack"; it will clarify his place in your home and it will win you the loyalty that he longs to lavish on you. With the gentle enforcement of regular boundaries, expressed through your words and gestures, you will raise a trusted friend.

In Conclusion

It is the nature of pets to look after their owners. Our commitment is to do the same. In their ongoing efforts to promote better pet care and to terminate animal neglect, the Humane Society of the United States suggests that pet owners take these actions:

1. Make sure your pet wears an identification tag so that he may be returned to you if lost.
2. To prevent destructive animal-behavioral problems, make sure you enroll your new puppy or dog in behavioral-training classes.
3. Animal behavioral problems can be health-related. Make sure your pet has a complete medical exam by a veterinarian at least once a year.
4. Prepare for disasters. Make sure you have a plan for your pet in the event of a hurricane, tornado, fire, or flood.
5. Plan for your pet's future in case something happens to you.
6. Learn how to avoid dog bites and how to prevent your dog from biting.
7. Make sure your pet is spayed or neutered.

Many people, in fact, are excellent pet owners, as illustrated in the following story. One day, an energetic black Lab named George ran out the front door of his owner's house. Charging across the street, he was seriously mauled by a car. The veterinarian said George would never walk again, but he stitched the mangled leg back in place nonetheless.

George's owner nursed him night and day, even obtaining permission from the doctor to sleep beside him overnight in the animal hospital as he lay recovering from a lengthy surgery. For many months, visiting neighbors would see them doing laps alongside each other in the swimming pool—physical therapy to strengthen George's damaged leg. "The ruined leg is now as strong and functional as the other, and you can't tell which one was injured," reports an incredulous veterinarian, who considers this case a miracle. The moral of the story is simply this: love heals.

Proper planning and preparation can lay the foundation for a priceless relationship with your pet. When a married couple who were considering children discussed the issue with their counselor, he advised against it, sensing their ambivalence. Likewise, instead of feeling that one "ought to" have pets, this is a decision, ideally, made with a sense of joy.

As one veterinarian commented when praised about her own pet, "He's not my dog; I'm his human."

Animals are easy members of the household or farm. You won't have to save for their college education, and they won't criticize your cooking. "Until one has loved an animal," noted the French novelist Anatole France, "a part of one's soul remains unawakened."

5

THE THEME ESSENCE FOR STRENGTH AND BALANCE

What is love? Is it only ours? Or does love whisper in the flowers?
J. Donald Walters

I want to present an exciting concept and a new way of looking at your pet through the eyes of his unique personality strengths. Like many animal enthusiasts, you may find this approach helpful in understanding your pets. We so love to identify and to understand them; following is a system to help you do just that.

Ego and Personality Defined

We might say someone has "a big ego," but we rarely hear an individual described as having "a big personality." To say "What an ego!" is considered unflattering, and yet saying "What a personality!" could be construed as quite a compliment. The term *ego* is defined as the individualized sense of I-ness that separates itself from its Source of life, or its higher, perfect Self. Ego also means our identification with a particular form, which also separates us from our higher, formless Self.

The main point here is separation. Much like an adolescent breaking away from his parents by affirming his identity as separate from them, the ego in man's nature establishes its individuation by pulling away from the Source of all life. The ego affirms, "I am a woman," or "I am a European." A certain level of self-consciousness, or self-awareness, is expressed in these statements.

The personality, however, is quite different from the ego. We could say that it is an offshoot of the ego. The personality is composed of the patterns, habits, likes, and dislikes, with their resulting desires, that lead a person to make specific choices. An example would be an individual saying, "I am a person with a love for justice, and therefore I want to devote my life to the study and practice of law." Here we see the person's likes and dislikes leading to a career choice that supports those desires.

How can we apply these definitions to the animal kingdom? We could say that animals have emerging egos, due to their entrapment in one or two *koshas* more than human beings. For instance, the wildebeest, a wild African antelope that lives in herds, has certain group characteristics. But no two gnus, as they are also called, are identical in personality. Animals are conscious beings, and they are conscious of life—but not self-conscious. Lower life forms, such as amoeba, may not be very far along in their expression of distinctive likes and dislikes, and thus their egos are not very strong. (I remember a cartoon portraying two amoeba sitting in their living room. The wife is comforting her husband by saying, "But Dear, you *are* the lowest form of life.")

Do plants have egos? The answer, looking at our evolutionary construct, would be no, unless we are talking about animated flowers in Disney cartoons. Plants have not yet separated themselves as individual egos, but they could be said to have a group expression, if not yet a group ego. Flowers do, however, express *qualities* of nature. It is precisely due to this lack of ego in the plant kingdom that plants embody such purity and power. We would see in them broad qualities of love or harmony or calmness rather than individuated expressions of these traits. It is these characteristics of the blossoms, in fact, that provide us with the healing art of flower essences.

Theme Essences Defined

For the last seventy years since the inception of the Bach Remedies, we have traditionally had only one word in the world of flower essences to describe essences in relation to personality: the *type* remedy. This term focuses on predominant negative qualities in the personality and labels a person or pet accordingly. For example, you might be described as a person who is picky and perfectionistic, with a strong sense of uncleanliness. Do any of us truly want to be defined in such negative terms?

The concept of theme essences, contrarily, identifies us and our animal friends through our fundamental personality strengths. A Cherry theme, by way of illustration, is undauntingly cheerful in all circumstances; a Lettuce theme is restfully calm. These terms apply beautifully to animals, for they are close to the plant world, and thus close to flower essences.

Our pets may be somewhat species- and/or breed-defined, but their developing personalities are nonetheless unmistakable. If you have a dachshund, for example—a German dog originally bred for badger hunting—you will notice in him the species characteristic of loyalty. This breed is known to be clever, courageous, and lively—all the qualities valued in a hunting dog. Thus, your dachshund, in particular, may be a Tomato or Corn theme. Within a particular breed, each individual animal expresses different subtleties of behavior and specific likes and dislikes that will override a breed-determined theme. As illustrated in the children's fable "The Tortoise and the Hare," you will rarely find a turtle with a Corn theme. Energy, as we know it, is not their hallmark! And yet Corn is a common theme for Abyssinian cats, who are noted for their agility, quickness, and constant desire to explore. Also, it may be more difficult to determine the theme essence of your goldfish than your goat; the higher the placement on the evolutionary ladder, the greater the expression of personality. Overall, animals express the pure qualities of nature represented in their theme essences with less interference from their minds and intellects than do people.

Wild animals are more likely to have theme essences and, likewise, personalities based on their breed, species, or both. The construct of theme essence, then, applies to the animal's unique personality that expresses greater definition through the very act of domestication. It is through ongoing contact with their human owners that these "personalities in process" develop in more individualized and unique ways. Domestication suggests, by definition, that animals no longer have to fend for themselves—to forage, to survive the elements and predators, and to reproduce. Their instinct for preservation can relax. In exchange, they must adapt to our strange world—whatever food we serve them, possibly a life indoors, and the inevitable issue of neutering, if we are sensitive to curbing the overpopulation and resultant euthanasia of millions of homeless animals.

Animals convey their personalities through their behavior just as people do. One dog left alone at home repeatedly for long periods of time might bark incessantly; another might tear up a rug; yet another, like Bonnet, mentioned in chapter 4, might mope and withdraw over time.

Molly, the cocker spaniel whose story is told in chapter 3, is a Raspberry theme. And whereas purebreds of any breed can become hyperactive and even neurotic by human standards, Molly is a perfect example of this theme's strengths. Befriending the young students, she is a loving companion for the children in her classroom, allowing them to cuddle and pet her, all the while exhibiting infinite patience. Molly's eyes are responsively lustrous; it appears as though she knows exactly what you are saying to her— a common trait for this theme. Raspberry themes are extremely sensitive. For this reason, Molly's abusive past deeply affected her on an emotional level. Had she been a Corn or a Pineapple theme—both stronger, more forcefully projected themes—she probably would have escaped the situation with less trauma.

How to Understand Your Pet's Theme Essence

How does the theme-essence concept apply to the treatment of animals through flower essences? The theme essence is the one that best matches the predominant positive quality in an animal's personality; it will be the essence that most balances him in his many and varied expressions: moods, habits, and preferences. If your pet seems "out of sorts," is fighting an illness, or is simply not acting like himself—administering his theme essence will help restore his equilibrium. Much as we grow by building on our existing strengths, animals do the same. And in a world—our domesticated world— to which they must adapt, their challenges are ongoing and many. The responses I receive about animals on their theme essence, and for people as well, is that taking this remedy is calming in a very gentle way.

How to determine your pet's theme essence? Observe him in a state of rest. Watch him at play. Notice how he interacts with other animals or members of your household. A childlike pet, even in advanced years, may be a Spinach theme, exhibiting simplicity and youthful qualities. A pet who seems older and wiser than his years but remains refreshingly inquisitive, by contrast, will be an Avocado theme.

If you still have difficulty determining your pet's theme essence, ask your children. Kids often have a wonderful ability to understand their dearly loved animal friends. Plus, their insights will generally not be as clouded as ours, with endless mental doubts, fears, and skepticism. You may overhear a child saying, "Oh, yes, Susie's a happy bird (Cherry)" or "My dog Robbie is really smart; he learned really fast how to stop jumping up on people (Avocado)."

Another excellent clue to determining your pet's theme essence is to observe what qualities he evokes in other pets and people. Back to our Cherry-theme animal: Here is a pet who cheers others in his environment. Likewise, the Corn theme energizes those around him. These principles apply to identifying theme essences for people as well. In addition, it is quite common to find a pet and owner who share the same theme.

Understanding theme essences also helps pet owners who are looking to successfully match a pet's theme with their own. Whereas like attracts like, as the saying goes, it is also true that opposites attract. See which of these truths applies to your own personality in adopting a pet. If you want a peaceful home, do not adopt a ferret, who will often be an energetic and enthusiastic Corn theme. On the other hand, if you are seeking a pet who will liven up your household, this species might be a very entertaining addition to your family. "Our ferret is a pretty fun little guy," one woman shared. "I kind of like him bouncing off the walls and dive-bombing my feet when I walk across the living room."

Human beings often possess not only a theme but a sub-theme as well. This means that one quality is particularly strong in the personality (the theme) and another is also predominant but slightly secondary (the sub-theme). Animals, both domesticated and wild, generally do not have sub-themes. Unlike people, they may exhibit a double theme. In this case, two positive personality qualities are identically strong and present in their natures. A lovebird, for instance, may be both cheerful (Cherry) and childlike (Spinach). Or a horse may be basically fearless (Tomato) and yet also express a deep compassion for his owner (Raspberry).

Please remember that we have generalized these concepts to some extent. Even an Avocado theme will possess some of the Corn theme's qualities and many, if not all, of the other flower essence strengths as well. And it is important to clarify that an animal need not be a Cherry-theme pet to exhibit the positive qualities of Cherry Essence. Hence, we may say that an animal could exhibit the positive Cherry state while at the same time having a different theme altogether. For the sake of clarity, though, these are the basic ideas to best assist you and your pets in their growth and overall happiness.

To summarize, then, animals and people grow in one of two ways: by enhancing existing strengths (theme) or by eliminating weaknesses (plot), which will be explained in the next chapter. Theme essences and plot essences are generic concepts that may be successfully applied to other flower essence lines as well.

How, then, can we use the construct of theme essences to help our pets? We can work with them better by understanding their strengths. Knowing that your Siamese cat is a Date theme, for example, you can tell her how sweet she is and reward her when she behaves in a manner in alignment with her theme essence. Or for an Avocado-theme dog, you might say, "Good for you! You remembered to bring in your toys!"

Theme Essences for Animals and Pet Owners

Here is a list of the twenty Master's Flower Essences and their identifying theme characteristics. (For a further explanation of this concept, and of plot essences in chapter 6, see *The Essential Flower Essence Handbook*.) Each essence is divided into two sections: one that defines the animal's theme personality and how he will influence his owner; the other, the owner's theme disposition and, in particular, how he will most likely care for his pet according to his theme-essence nature. This section also illustrates how well-matched a pet and same-theme owner can be. It is designed to help you understand and care for your pets more insightfully. You may want to see which of these themes apply to you and your animal companions.

Almond-Theme Animals: Self-control

The animal who lives a quiet life and is balanced and moderate in his eating and sleeping habits and other daily activities is an Almond theme. His is a calming presence—unobtrusive in the household, and yet always there. Visitors to the home may say, "Oh, I didn't know he was here!" Some animals thoroughly dominate a home with their personalities. The Almond-theme pet's personality is so inward that his presence is not experienced in an imposing way.

Paradoxically, although you may not sense his presence, you will feel his absence. His behavior may go unnoticed; he has no need to draw attention to himself through noise or destruction of property. He is, basically, content within himself and balanced in the expression of his needs. He will not place demands on you.

This pet offers an example of nature's quality of a calming stillness. When undisturbed by man-made intrusions such as pollution, traffic, or clear-cutting, Nature is at peace with herself, much like the Almond-theme animal. Nature epitomizes moderation and balanced living, as does this quiet pet.

Almond-Theme Pet Owners: Self-control

The Almond-theme owner is practically inconspicuous in his own home. He tends to spend a lot of time around the house, which is a plus for house pets who enjoy the companionship of their human friend. This theme owner is easy to be around and comfortable to live with. He may be married, and happily so, but will not at all mind remaining single. Moderate in his habits, he is generally an early-to-bed-early-to-rise person. The television will not be turned up too loud—if he ever watches it—and he is not one for throwing wild parties. His home is a perfect haven for pets.

This household, reflective of its Almond-theme owner, will be tidy with everything in its place. It may be impressive but not lavishly decorated, and it will be functional. Space will be wisely used without much clutter. Pets will be accommodated both with furniture to nap on (if allowed or appropriate) and areas to run around a bit.

This pet owner takes good care of his animals, respecting their need for regularity and routine. Himself a quiet individual, his pets will readily absorb his calmness. The almond tree itself symbolizes the quality of moderation in its height; its trunk is neither tall nor short. This sense of balance rather than extremes characterizes the Almond-theme pet owner as well. He will share his home comfortably and quietly with his pets, providing them with a fortifying environment in which to grow.

Apple-Theme Animals: Healthfulness

The animal who loves to race, swim, gallop, or explore the possibilities of movement simply for the joy of it is most likely an Apple theme. He is alert and basically "bright-eyed and bushy-tailed." A certain glow to his physical body radiates from his innate joy in being in this world. If we could read the Apple-theme animal's mind, it would be free of the worry, fear, and doubt that so often plague his human companions. Note: It may seem easy at first to confuse this theme animal with Corn; to clarify, the Apple theme is generally not as physically active as the Corn theme and spends more time at rest.

The Apple-theme animal is good-natured and tends to not fret. More often than not, he has come from a healthy home free from neglect, abuse, or improper training. Chances are that he was not weaned too early and basically got off to a good, functional start.

Your Apple-theme companion is ready to accompany you on an exercise routine at a moment's notice. A workout is important for him; it is a basic way that he expresses himself and lets off steam.

Even when ill, the Apple-theme pet will seem OK and mainly unaffected by infirmity, more so than other animals. His basic personality is so health-oriented that a serious illness or accident will not affect him the way it would other animals. This pet is deeply inspiring to his owner for his natural ability to exemplify health and what is required to possess it. His attitudes and actions alike provide a blueprint for a robust relationship between pet and owner.

Apple-Theme Pet Owners: Healthfulness

The health nut or sports enthusiast exemplifies the Apple-theme owner's basic personality. Even if he is not particularly physically active, he will understand the elements of health: proper diet, exercise, fresh air, and moderate amounts of sunlight, meditation, and wholesome company. He will be aware of blood pressure and cholesterol issues. This individual may be well-versed in different health regimens or the latest nutritional recommendations.

The blush of the apple blossom, a vibrant white flower accented with shades of pink, glows in the Apple theme's complexion. He will have the inner stamina of a long-distance runner and the commitment to health of a trained nutritionist. This theme individual is not a sports spectator but a full participant.

Understanding the importance of proper diet, hygiene, and nutrition, his pets will receive the same care he allots to himself. His concern about diet will ensure that they receive food minus the harmful, toxic additives so often contained in pet products these days. He will use nontoxic household cleansers and most of all will provide adequate floor or yard space for his animal's comfort and health. And his pets will get plenty of exercise.

Even as apples are hardy trees that thrive on a wide range of soils, the Apple-theme pet owner radiates this quality to his pets. Animals in this home will be healthy, balanced pets who are especially easy to train and tend to recover well from illness—just like their owner.

Avocado-Theme Animals: Good memory

The Avocado-theme pet is ever alert and lives fully in the moment, even more than most animals. He is inquisitive and curious, always exploring, and eager to learn more about his environment and those with whom he shares it. Animals, as a rule, live in the present rather than being scattered over the past and future as human beings often are. Thus they are able to deeply feel, sense, and perceive their daily experiences.

The Avocado-theme animal responds to proper training more quickly than other animals. Since he will remember what he is taught, any "memory lapses" on his part are a statement that he is somehow upset and the issue at hand needs to be attended to. An Avocado-theme cat, for example, who soils outside the litter box is insisting on your awareness of the current problem—which probably has something to do with you, the owner (see chapter 4).

This pet is very responsive to your verbal and nonverbal messages alike. He will generally return home when called. Even in infancy or childhood, the Avocado-theme animal has the temperament of one much older. If you have the opportunity to see him with his siblings, he will stand out for his maturity, seeming wiser than his years—or weeks, as the case may be—even though he lacks experience to validate his sophistication. He may still be a colt or a puppy, but he will seem to know what's going on more than the others in his immediate animal family.

A genuine sparkle will be added to your household through this animal's presence. It is a good idea before bringing him home to be certain of a workable matching of personalities so that his inquisitiveness—common among all animals but accentuated in this theme—is a good match with others in the home.

Avocado-Theme Pet Owners: Good memory

The inventor, the scientist, the bookworm—these titles apply to the mental state of an Avocado-theme owner. An avid interest in learning characterizes his temperament. A wonderful owner for the more inquisitive animal species and breeds, this theme's pets will find a world of new experiences in this household as well as a kindred spirit in their owner.

As a potential pet owner, an Avocado-theme individual will study, read, inquire, and surf Web sites to learn all he can about his potential pets. Any animals who are brought into his home have indeed been well researched beforehand! His joy in gathering knowledge about their origins, unusual facts, behavioral traits, and specific needs is outweighed only by his interest in integrating them comfortably into his household.

The Avocado-theme owner has a tremendously focused mind and thus provides very uplifting company for his animals. His alertness rallies their own innate ability to live in the present moment. This owner is a natural communicator with the animal kingdom. His ability to concentrate his mind, pick up subtle behavioral clues, and read a pet's body language allows for a natural rapport between pet and pet owner.

Mentally astute and inventive, the Avocado theme will benefit from the earthy balance of sharing his home with animals. If they too are explorers, many good times in the home and field will be had by all.

Banana-Theme Animals: Humility

The Banana-theme pet is about as easy to get along with as a pet can be. He makes a wonderful addition to any household for this very reason. Exceedingly accommodating to other animals, he will graciously bow out of any hissing matches or claiming-of-territory battles. Gentle and humble, the Banana-theme pet is often overlooked, somewhat like the Almond-theme animal. This pet, however, knows how to look after himself. His needs are minimal, and he will tend not to balk if routines, such as feeding times, are tardy.

This pet is calm and thus calming to be around. While he is not assertive by nature, neither is he the "house doormat." Rather than defending himself, he will defend property. If a dog, this theme animal will not bark so much for attention as to protect his owner and property. Even highly vocal animals of this nature may seem to retain an air of calm quietude.

The Banana-theme animal will tend to let children roughhouse with him to an extraordinary degree without getting ruffled. Enormously patient with them, he seems to enjoy group activities more through the joy of others involved. Banana-theme animals will enter and exit your life with an unmistakable sense of calmness. Consider yourself fortunate to own, and be owned by, this animal!

Banana-Theme Pet Owners: Humility

The Banana-theme owner will be unusually kind and gentle. He will share his home easily with people and pets alike; no toes, or paws, will be stepped on. Due to a basic lack of identification with his own ego, to a greater or lesser extent, he does not view his home as "his" but rather as a dwelling place that is shared by all. He creates a refreshingly unemotional atmos-phere; personality conflicts with pets or other people will be minimal. After all, what has he to defend?

As a result, the atmosphere of this theme's property will be relaxed. He will raise healthy pets who will absorb their owner's lack of self-absorption. He will enjoy his animals dearly but in an impersonal way. People of this theme are fairly aware of their own littleness, so to speak, within the bigger picture. They will not impose their moods, likes, or dislikes on their animals. Their attitudes foster a pervasive calmness throughout the household.

The Banana-theme owner will see that all of his animal friends' needs are met, and he is not given to playing favorites. Each and every pet will sense an important place in this home, even those animals who are more territorial and hierarchy-oriented by nature. In this humble home, calmness reigns.

Blackberry-Theme Animals: Purity

The Blackberry-theme pet possesses a certain innocence and lack of guile. He may be sleek in appearance or exhibit other physical characteristics reflective of his personality. He will seem to be very aware of his environment and those with whom he shares it. A knowing look gleams in his eyes—perhaps because he actually does know what's going on. He makes a trusting companion, one you may feel you can talk to and share your thoughts with—as though you have gone to see an excellent therapist. Articulate though not imposing in making his needs known, this pet is a loving companion with whom you can have a multifaceted relationship. He will also radiate a certain maturity, and you may at times forget that he is not human!

Basically, depending somewhat on the species, the Blackberry-theme pet will be a very clean animal. If a dog, he can be easily trained to put his toys away; if a cat, there will be few, if any, litter-box issues in the household, barring physical symptoms and owner-induced problems. Grooming—by himself and you—is important to this theme animal. In fact, brushing, preening, and primping are wonderful ways to relate to him.

The Blackberry-theme animal, especially if a cat, will appear to be offended by any untidiness in the household. He will find stepping in a dollop of jam on the kitchen floor not at all to his liking. Furthermore, it is better not to leave shoes, umbrellas, or other objects lying around that will disturb his "space." Cats are largely aware of their environment much as an extension of themselves, and they do prefer to have everything in order.

Blackberry-Theme Pet Owners: Purity

Blackberry themes tend to be principled, well-educated, and profoundly insightful people. The wild blackberry bush, a member of the rose family, grows low to the ground on thorny vines and produces delicate lavender-white blossoms. Reflecting the characteristics of this fruit-bearing bush, the Blackberry theme possesses an ability to see into the heart of issues, which makes them excellent therapists and counselors or simply good friends with whom you can talk about your problems.

A Blackberry-theme owner paired with a same-theme pet is indeed a perfect match. This owner, much like his animal, prefers "a place for everything and everything in its place." Purity and cleanliness, in thoughts and living space alike, are the qualities by which he lives.

He will speak to his pet as though to another human being; in fact, the pet may seem to respond accordingly. This owner has a kindly sense of humor as well as an innate dislike of negativity and dishonesty in others. His pets will benefit from his straightforwardness. No ambivalent training methods will be employed by this owner; he is as good as his word.

Cherry-Theme Animals: Cheerfulness

If animals could sing and dance, Cherry themes would do so. Highly entertaining, they will cheer you and make you laugh with their antics and frolicking. You may find yourself watching less television or renting fewer videos with a Cherry-theme pet in your home! And although all young animals will frequently exhibit both Cherry- and Spinach-theme characteristics, their actual theme essence may be altogether different.

The cheery, Cherry-theme nature is not to be confused with a frantic or frenetic personality, because they are basically even-tempered and easygoing. These themes remain youthful throughout their lives; nothing appeals to them more than a good game, a tickle, or a scratch behind the ears, no matter how old they are. Light-footed, they will tend to prance rather than walk.

You will find in them both a playfulness and a more watchful behavior. They enjoy being participants as well as spectators when it comes to lively activities. For although they like to play—and may even seem to live for it—they also know how to pull back and not physically exhaust themselves. Theirs is a rich yet light nature; their companionship provides the owner, including children, with sincere friends who can quietly retreat when necessary. These animals are not prone to moods. They will be consistently cheerful and dependably good-natured.

The Cherry-theme pet has much to offer his human friends. Although he may not have to trudge off to work every day like his human companions, he does his "work" around the house or yard with an even temperament, look-ing after other animals on the property or overseeing and protecting the home. With proper training, he is especially good with, and for, children.

Cherry-Theme Pet Owners: Cheerfulness

The Cherry-theme owner, somewhat like the Spinach theme, is very childlike. Lighthearted and bubbly by nature, this individual places a high priority on having a good time. His speech is filled with laughter, smiles, and jokes. Others feel lighter in his presence. If you've had a hard day, spend time with this theme. If you're caught in a mood, being in his presence will help it to lift noticeably or evaporate altogether.

The Cherry-theme owner may not have the tidiest home or yard, but a spirit of fun will prevail. He likes to connect with people and animals, as his joy is contagious and he is all for sharing it, sometimes in the form of the latest joke he has heard. At the same time, a level of even-mindedness underlies this theme's personality. He is even-keeled as well as good-natured. This owner will also appreciate a certain element of impersonality with his pets. Although these two sides to his character may seem paradoxi-cal, they offer a wonderful stability to his overall nature, making him a delightful pet owner. His pets will tend to be happy and well-balanced.

This individual is a perfect match for rambunctious, lively, and playful animals. He will be romping right alongside them. In fact, it may be diffi-cult to tell who is having more fun—the pet or the Cherry-theme owner. Ferrets as a species provide endless rounds of fun for this owner. He also relates well to young animals who, regardless of breed or species, are more lively than their elders. Older animals belonging to this theme owner will act and feel younger in a Cherry home. Because of his own "Cherryness," this person will awaken the playful side in his pets. And what a lively household this is!

Coconut-Theme Animals: Upliftment

Coconut-theme pets make wonderful companions. Coconut themes are one of the more challenging kind to detect through behavioral clues, but we can make a few generalizations about them. They tend to be very bright and uncommonly alert. Much as an Avocado-theme pet may look older than his years, the Coconut-theme animal often appears to know more than he lets on.

Coconut themes seem able to transcend difficult situations in very impressive ways. They can adapt readily to infirmities and deal especially well with their creaking bodies as they age. They tend to get along with other animals in the household, even if their species or breed as a whole would generally have difficulty. In fact, we could say that this animal is one who basically transcends hardships very well.

Deeply committed to their owners and environments, these pets possess a certain stamina. They will weather illness and injury better than most other animals. They will also persevere until they learn the behaviors taught to them by their owner.

Coconut-Theme Pet Owners: Upliftment

Coconut-theme owners are always looking for better ways to do things—not as much in mundane ways of improving on existing data but more in terms of finding solutions to problems. One would be inclined to call these people great thinkers; however, they do not access their answers from the level of thought. Coconut themes are problem-solvers. A simple example follows. When it rains, an outdoor landscaper who cannot work in such conditions finds other productive ways to use his time, such as designing an installation and researching where to purchase the necessary plants, sod, and materials for the job. Thus he finds a solution to his problem; in fact, he finds an answer within the actual context of the obstacle itself.

Applying this concept to their role as pet owners, these themes are always looking for better ways to raise their pets. Their concern is to give their animals the best possible care. When a Coconut-theme owner spends time with his pet, it is done with awareness. This does not mean he is a constant disciplinarian or a rigid taskmaster. His interest is in spending "quality time" with his animal companion—sharing a walk in the sunshine, going for a ride in the country, or singing harmonies with his bird perched on his shoulder, all with the expressed intent of developing a deeper relationship with his pet.

The Coconut-theme owner values bonding with his animals. He knows that he has much to learn from them and that each animal in his home can be a way for him to connect more deeply with the animal kingdom in its entirety as well as with Nature herself.

Corn-Theme Animals: Vitality

The Corn-theme pet is characterized by three qualities: energy, energy, and energy! Enthusiastic and joyful, he is raring to go for new experiences. Unlike some animals who are afraid to try anything outside their normal routine or to go to places that are unfamiliar to them, this animal is quite an adventurer. He welcomes new experiences rather than shrinking from them.

Even older animals of this theme will remain energetic throughout their lives. They amaze their human friends on a regular basis with their endless interest in new escapades. Finding different ways to perform their regular activities, even hamsters in their cages will invent innovative routines for spinning on their wheels.

Greater energy levels breed contented pets. You won't find a lethargic animal, unless old or infirm, who seems happy. The Corn-theme pet, on the other hand, races across a cage, lawn, or field with tremendous enthusiasm. Whatever his physical display of exercise, it exudes an abundant joy. Here we see the sheer delight of an animal exploring his physical abilities and new environs at the same time. If your Corn-theme canine could speak, he might say, "It is a good day to be a dog!"

Corn-Theme Pet Owners: Vitality

The Corn-theme owner mirrors the Corn-theme pet in practically every aspect. As a corn stalk grows best with plenty of sunlight, this theme owner flourishes with positive bursts of energy. He will not allow himself to feel blocked by negative thought patterns. Procrastination is not likely an attribute of his personality. "If you want something done," the saying goes, "ask a busy person." Or, one might add, ask a Corn theme.

For this reason, the Corn theme makes a very fine pet owner. He is always thinking up new ways to make his home or land more comfortable for his pets—a bit like the Coconut theme, but with great energy to himself do the building or remodeling. Similar to the Apple theme, he enjoys exercising and sharing activities with his animals. A good jog on the beach or a ride in the country are favorite pastimes for him. The pets of this owner will rarely find themselves bored!

The Corn-theme owner will often rearrange furniture, bring new art pieces home, change the decor, and make improvements on his outdoor facilities as well. Were it not for the consistency of his energy, this household would be destabilizing for his pets. As the Corn theme's profuse vitality is anchored in great joy, he creates an entertaining environment for his pets.

Date-Theme Animals: Sweetness, tenderness

This animal will strike a special chord in your heart for his sweetness in the way he relates to others and to you. His behavior will include many actions that are endearing and richly expressive of a deeply loving animal. The Date-theme animal will match the Peach-theme pet for the embracing nature of his actions. Also similar to the Grape theme in his outpouring of loving expression, the Date theme will make you feel, through myriad gestures, that you are "the cat's meow."

Much as the date fruit possesses a sweetness as satisfying as the richest chocolate, this pet will sweeten your life again and again. You may find yourself following him around with a camera to capture the many special moments in which he will express sheer beauty through his silently loving personality. It may be categorically said that all animals possess an abundance of Date's sweetness, for it is not within their natures to judge, criticize, or compare. For these qualities alone, we can fully open ourselves to our pets without fear of rebuke.

Other animals and people often want to befriend this pet. Neighbors, family members, friends, and even strangers will all notice something special about your Date-theme animal companion. You'll find yourself commenting of this pet many times, "Oh, how sweet!"

Date-Theme Pet Owners: Sweetness, tenderness

The Date-theme owner also excels in the quality of acceptance of others. He is a "safe" person to have as a friend due to his utter lack of negative judgment. Being sweet himself, he will tend to see sweetness in others. This individual is not easily irritated, nor does he provoke discomfort— a quality that often accompanies individuals of sour disposition. He makes friends readily and loves to have company visit, which can be a treat for his pets as well.

Pets of this theme will feel more than fed and sheltered; they will feel embraced. Through the Date theme's voice and eyes especially, his pets will know nurturing, never harshness. This theme feeds his animals with tenderness, and he cleans the barn or litter box in that same spirit.

The Date-theme pet owner loves to express this sweetness through buying both practical and frivolous presents for his animal friends. And if the household shelters multiple pets, each one will have his own toys or food bowls. Everyone is treated with tenderness in the Date theme's home.

Fig-Theme Animals: Flexibility

Here is an animal who remains relaxed under all circumstances. Somewhat like the Grape theme, the Fig-theme pet accepts the presence of other pets in the household, though based on his own easygoing attitudes rather than the Grape theme's deep love. He also makes friends easily and generally seems very comfortable with himself. His comfort is not to be mistaken for laziness; it merely represents a certain flow to his personality.

The Fig-theme pet is very flexible; he can either follow routines or just as easily alter the course of the day. As a rule, he tends to travel well. A break in the normal schedule will not upset him as it would other animals. He doesn't seem to mind waiting if meals are served late—though it is always a good idea to tend to the cleaning of his living area and location of evacuation. (For animals such as goats and cows who must be milked on a daily basis, however, regularity for the sake of their health is paramount.)

Perhaps the most special quality of the Fig-theme animal is the way that others begin to feel more comfortable about themselves in his presence. People may laugh more often around him, though never at him. Laughter and good humor derive from a lack of rigidity in people and their pets. And this adaptable theme animal enjoys a good laugh with the best of them.

Fig-Theme Pet Owners: Flexibility

Fig-theme owners tend to be fluid in both their body language and their attitudes. One of their favorite words is "Whatever." This characteristic is not a sign of weakness but rather of great strength. They can adapt to people and places easily, and they make wonderful travelers and traveling companions. They are open to new experiences and are comfortable in any number of different environments.

Animals feel especially at home with a Fig-theme pet owner or animal lover. They instinctively sense his easygoing nature and are instantly set at ease in his presence. As the Fig Essence is used to help soften too strict a sense of discipline, the Fig-theme individual is extremely accommodating by nature. He will be able to blend his own quirks and idiosyncrasies easily with his animals and readily adapt to theirs as well.

Grape-Theme Animals: Love, devotion

The Grape-theme animal is the pet among pets for his ability to love. Much like the Apple theme, he most likely enjoyed a very healthy infancy without being weaned from his mother or separated from siblings too early. He tends to adjust quite nicely to other pets in the household, even if he belongs to a species such as cats that typically has difficulty in this situation. Jealousy, neediness, clinging, and bullying behavior are generally not symptoms of this theme's personality.

This animal expresses deep loyalty and devotion to his owners and to other animals. He will be a lifelong friend, constant in the expression of his commitment to you, your family, and your property. He relates well to people and animals of all ages without feeling threatened by them. As a Grape-theme pet possesses a certain fullness to his personality, your home will feel somehow full when he lives there. Even if he is an "only pet," he will transform it from a house to a home.

With a Grape theme in your life, you will never feel alone. His presence will fill your home and heart alike. One word of caution: The passing of this pet may be very difficult for the owner, and the grieving process may take some time. As this pet's dearness is keenly felt throughout his lifetime, he will be acutely missed when he is gone. In chapter 7, "When a Pet Dies,"

I offer some suggestions, including flower essences and their applications, to help the pet owner.

Grape-Theme Pet Owners: Love, devotion

Grape-theme owners are, simply, loving people. Grape themes connect especially well with their animals, for they love their pets as their pets love them. They love without condition. They love freely. Their love does not have to be earned; it is simply bestowed. For this reason alone, people and pets love them in return.

The Grape-theme individual, regardless of age, relates deeply to others no matter how old they are. These people intuit that pure love is completely free of personal need, desire, or a sense of lack. They understand that, even when a loved one leaves or passes away, love is never lost.

Animals in the care of a Grape-theme individual will feel nurtured, accepted, and befriended. These people make especially good owners for previously abandoned, neglected, or abused animals. Pets who have been badly treated oftentimes need special care and understanding for their behavioral problems, symptomatic of poor treatment. Grape-theme owners possess the intuitive understanding and resultant patience necessary to care for these special creatures. They know, as the old Beatles song goes, that "All you need is love."

Lettuce-Theme Animals: Calmness

The Lettuce-theme pet is a calm animal with a strongly felt presence. Whereas the Almond-theme animal is also calm, he may not be noticed in the household until he is absent. The Lettuce theme, conversely, makes himself known, but in a very comforting way. Not to be mistaken with lazy, this pet is a storehouse of energy. However, there is a certain quietness about him, with no sense of demand or need. Energetic but not hasty in his actions, he will touch your heart with his depth and lightness at the same time.

This pet will communicate his needs and wants to you in a quiet, almost telepathic way. You may find that somehow you "just know" what he is trying to get across to you. Individuals to whom communication is important will find a very rewarding relationship with this particular theme animal.

The Lettuce-theme pet may even appear contemplative or reflective at times. His movements will be soft, as though his paws or hooves do not quite touch the ground. He is gentle with other pets in the household or on the land, as though he communicates with them in silent ways as well. Being in his presence will make you more aware of your own calmness—or lack of it. His quiet demeanor will remind you to not waste your energy in restless and nervous activities. This theme makes a wonderful companion.

Lettuce-Theme Pet Owners: Calmness

Lettuce-theme owners are quiet but not shy, retiring but not boring. In fact, they tend to be highly creative. As they also excel in the art of communicating their thoughts and feelings, they will often say things in innovative ways. They make excellent writers. They tend to speak little, but when they do, others listen.

A Lettuce-theme individual will be calming to his friends and family, especially when they are troubled or emotionally agitated. As an owner of animals, this theme will also be a great comfort to his pets. He tends to not get upset over discipline problems, litter-box accidents, or wear and tear on his property. To him, nothing is worth the price of lost calmness, and everything is fixable.

Orange-Theme Animals: Joy

If pets could smile, Orange themes would do so. These animals possess an infinite capacity to enjoy this world in as many ways as possible. They love to explore the movement of their bodies. They enjoy new places as well as old. They are happy when visitors come to their home. Their joy runs deep. You might find yourself wanting to ask them, "What are you so happy about?" They just are.

These animals will provide special companionship when their owners are grieving or depressed. To some extent, as animals do, they will absorb the sadness of their owners. Even then, these theme pets will be able to retain their own sense of happiness and basically remain untouched by any despair in the home.

Orange themes, both human and animal, have a certain resilience in their personalities and an ability to bounce back, as it were, from even the deepest sorrow. Much as the orange tree, a small evergreen, grows in regions where frosts are virtually unknown, sadness is a quality relatively unfamiliar to this theme animal.

Orange-Theme Pet Owners: Joy

Unlike the Cherry-theme individual with his bubbly lightness, the Orange-theme owner's joy is very deep. The Cherry theme's signature is his laughter; the Orange theme's is his smile. Often, though not always, this individual has actually had a very hard life with repeated difficulties and challenges. Through it all, he has kept hold of an inner joy that carries him through the worst of times.

These themes provide special testimony to the concept that our theme essence is based on who we are and not on what we do—that it is who we are which sustains us through the events that befall us as we move through our experiences in this world. Pertaining to the Orange theme, this person, through repeated opportunities to grow and make choices, *becomes* the joy of his theme essence.

Even though some animals, such as cats, do not at all enjoy the scent of citrus, they will usually adore the Orange-theme pet owner. Joy is a contagious quality; animals readily sense its presence. Pets tune in to a certain joyful fullness in the Orange theme's personality, much like the roundness of a perfectly ripe orange fruit.

Animals who live in an Orange theme's household are very happy pets. Their needs are met far beyond the basic level of food and shelter. Food is served with joy; bedding is prepared with a gladness in being able to provide for them.

Peach-Theme Animals: Selflessness

The Peach-theme pet is a truly selfless animal. These animals are the care-takers of their caregivers, and they tend to act in mothering ways with other pets as well. "Born nurturers" defines the Peach-theme animal. He senses when others are unwell or emotionally troubled and gives them energy. You may often find him grooming other pets in the household or expressing his care for them through a variety of demonstrative behaviors.

This theme loves to share his toys or include his fellow housemates in his games. He is an especially good pet to have with children, as he will always seem to be looking out for them as well.

If others in the home, either human or animal, are struggling with emotional issues or are physically unwell, the Peach-theme pet will be giving his energy where it is needed. As the Peach-theme owner will intuit his animal's needs, so the Peach-theme pet tunes in to the needs of those in the home. He may come and sit by you or give you a special nudge. Whatever the form, he is giving you the deepest nurturing love from his trusting heart. A better friend in this world is hard to find.

Peach-Theme Pet Owners: Selflessness

Each of the twenty pet-theme owners possesses a special quality expressive of his skills as an animal's guardian, Peach being no exception. The gentleness of this theme individual and his natural ability to communicate and commune with his animals is quietly extraordinary. Much as the mother knows the needs of her children even before they express them, so the Peach-theme pet owner understands his animals. This owner can often sense when his pet is feeling under the weather and may need changes in his diet or living quarters before any outer signs appear.

Peach-theme individuals, personifying this mothering essence, are always taking care of the needs of others before their own. Rather than being depleted by their ministrations, they are energized. Their joy lies in serving others. Their special gift is knowing that others are an extension of their own being and that in serving others, they are served as well.

Many studies have been conducted on the power of prayer. Reports unanimously confirm that the person praying receives an even greater benefit than the individual for whom he is praying. In a sense, we could say that a Peach-theme owner's care for his pet is a form of constant prayer, expressed through his concern for the animal's welfare. A pet in this household will be well tended and very well loved.

Pear-Theme Animals: Peacefulness

The Pear-theme pet is a healer. You'll find yourself just wanting to "hang around" him. Being with him will be a calming experience, as he holds a special place among all theme animals of the Master's Essences line. This pet is the equivalent, in animal form, of our Emergency Essence. Steady in nature, balanced and unflappable, the Pear-theme pet is a source of comfort to all. He handles himself especially well in a crisis. In addition, he can endure illness or injury to his own body with quiet equanimity, more so than most animals, somewhat like Apple and Coconut themes. It is a good idea, however, to properly assess the severity of his condition and call on veterinary care if necessary, as he deals so well with symptoms that their urgency or seriousness may be overlooked.

It is safe to generalize in saying that all animals are born with an intrinsic connection to Nature. Were it not for our domestication of them, Nature would be their source of food, shelter, companionship, and lastly, their demise. But the Pear-theme pet's link with nature is many times stronger than in other animals. As a result of this deeper connection, his instinctive nature and resultant intuition will be heightened. More so than most animals, he will sense changes in the weather; he will anticipate calamities, both natural and man-made; and he will basically be an accurate barometer of impending events.

This pet is a great gift to any household. His innate peacefulness will positively affect the energy of any children in the home who are typically wound up, and he will calm the adults as well. In general, his energy will tend to pacify them, rather than their agitation affecting him.

Many shelters and pounds are filled with Pear-theme animals waiting to contribute their peaceful presence to homes throughout the world. These are the pets by whom you will find yourself permanently changed, possibly many years after their passing.

Pear-Theme Pet Owners: Peacefulness

Pear-theme owners are, to use a slang word, mellow. They create comfortable homes in which people and animals can let their guard down and deeply relax. If valuables are broken by their pets, it's OK. If messes happen on the floor, that's fine too. These theme owners understand that the true valuables in their home are the pets and people who occupy it. In fact, you may often hear them repeat the words, "It's OK; don't worry about it."

If you visit a Pear theme's home when you are tired, you will find yourself feeling rested. Arriving in a state of tightly wound anxiety, you will find yourself able to slow down. Much as the pear tree grows in temperate climates and needs little tending, this theme is solid, firmly rooted, and deeply linked to Nature's healing rhythms.

Pear themes who take on the responsibility of pets have no trouble integrating them into their lives. These themes relate to anything earthy, including members of the mineral and plant kingdoms as well as the animal kingdom. Oftentimes, the decor of their homes will include rock work or clay pottery, lush plants that cover counter space and window ledges, and a wonderful array of animals. Many times, they will have more than one breed or species in their home, all of them generally compatible and accepting of each other.

Pineapple-Theme Animals: *Self-assuredness*

The Pineapple-theme pet loves to be the center of attention and expresses a genuine and innocent pride in his accomplishments, almost as if saying, "Look what I can do!" Cats who proudly bring home a mouse or bird for their owner are expressing, to some extent, the qualities of the Pineapple theme. The dog who seems pleased with his ability to successfully keep intruders off his owner's property does likewise.

A charmer and a show-stopper, this is the pet we can't keep our eyes off of. He may be extremely attractive with an eye-catchingly healthy coat or majestic plume, or there may be something particularly attention-getting in his body language.

In any case, the Pineapple-theme pet seems well on his way to developing a strong sense of his own identity. This animal often exhibits idiosyncrasies. You may find yourself spellbound at his antics. He also likes to show off when company visits, sometimes with a knowing gleam in his eye. He will find your lavish praise at these times healthy and affirming.

These animals tend to be very intelligent, and when they begin expressing strong likes and dislikes and various preferences about their surroundings, we may clearly recognize the sprouting seeds of personality.

Pineapple-Theme Pet Owners: Self-assuredness

The Pineapple-theme owner loves to be the life of the party, even when no party is happening. Sometimes eccentric, and glaringly so, the Pineapple theme is clearly an individualist. He forms very distinctive ideas on many subjects, and his laughter will ring out in a gathering of people. Charismatic by nature, he tends to stand out in a crowd.

Spending time in the company of a Pineapple theme is exuberantly refreshing. He infuses those around him with a healthy self-assuredness. Never a doormat, neither is he overbearing.

The Pineapple-theme owner tends to draw into his household or create animals with individual temperaments. Valuing his own individuality, he respects the same in his pets. They will feel free to express their particular preferences in games, food, and toys. He enjoys making each pet feel very special and deeply appreciated.

Raspberry-Theme Animals: Kindheartedness

A more kindhearted animal is not to be found. A friend, a comforter, and a very sensitive pet with a highly sensitized feeling nature, this animal is good with people of all ages, especially children. We might say that the Raspberry-theme pet is good at "reading" people's energy. If you see him walk boldly up to a stranger and roll at his feet as a sign of trust or bravely sniff him out, you may safely assume that the person is himself kindly. Contrarily, if you see your Raspberry-theme pet shying away, hissing, or growling at someone for no apparent reason, that person may be of shady character.

Raspberry-theme pets bond deeply with their owners who, in turn, find in them the closest of friends. Here is a pet who readily makes eye contact with you. His eyes will tend to be expressive and responsive. Quite often, you will see something recognizably human in them—that quality coined as "the milk of human kindness."

People fortunate enough to have Raspberry-theme pets in their household frequently say that they feel they can talk to them. Not only will you find yourself talking aloud to these pets, but you may have the sense that they are listening—and understanding as well. Best of all, they will not judge, blame, or lecture on the subject of your faults. Who can be a truer friend?

Raspberry-Theme Pet Owners: Kindheartedness

Raspberry-theme individuals are noted for their far-reaching kindheartedness, embracing all living things with their compassion. These people are sensitive, sympathetic, and empathetic. Listening is one of their natural gifts. Most of all, they understand the various emotional wounds that people and pets can suffer—specifically, feeling hurt, holding grudges, and bouts of anger that stem from contained emotional pain. Even though animals live fully in each moment, they can also exhibit negative behaviors stemming from emotional damage much like people; a visit with a Raspberry theme, similar to taking Raspberry Essence, may be "just what the doctor ordered."

Raspberry themes make ideal pet owners. Their innate compassion extends easily to their pets. They are always concerned and caring. Far and beyond their pets' physical needs, they will want to be certain that their animals are happy in the homes they create. They tend to empathetically feel their pet's pain.

These owners understand the rhythms of their pets—when they want company, when they want rest, when they need special attention, or when something upsets them. They can also understand that disturbed or inappropriate behavior may stem from past abuse rather than improper training. For this reason, these people—both similar to and different from Grape themes—make especially good owners for animals who have been mistreated.

Spinach-Theme Animals: Simplicity

The best word to describe a Spinach-theme pet is "delightful." The eternal child-animal, this pet will embody the qualities of innocence and trust throughout his entire lifetime. Even in later years, he will remain playful and fun-loving. A special gleam in his eye says it's always time to play and every-thing is a game. This is the animal who will approach you with a toy or two in his mouth, drop it at your feet, and sit quietly looking at you, waiting for you to, literally, "take the ball and run with it." His message is simple: He wants to play.

Spinach-theme animals are easygoing in a manner different from the Pear theme, whose relaxation stems from a deeper connection with nature than most animals. The Spinach theme's sense of ease is based on his abil-ity to trust, as do children, that everything will be taken care of and that they have no need to worry. These animals are basically stress-free.

For this reason, Spinach-theme pets are very soothing to nervous own-ers. Their mere presence in a household helps everyone to lighten up. And with modern-day tensions at an all-time high as we enter a new millen-nium—an unstable economy, political unrest, and the hovering possibility of warfare—a Spinach-theme animal in the household is practically a nec-essary addition.

Spinach-Theme Pet Owners: Simplicity

The Spinach-theme owner, himself childlike, likes to have fun. Playful by nature, much like the Spinach-theme pet, he is always ready for a good joke, a fun game, or a spontaneous trip to the zoo. In fact, these people will often laugh the loudest at their own jokes. Even as an adult, he will probably enjoy cartoons and children's movies for their message of simplicity, which is his special hallmark.

People sense the Spinach theme's straightforwardness and find him trustworthy. He is not given to dishonesty and, in fact, is not very good at all at lying. The delicate yellow blossoms of the quickly maturing spinach plant grow in the juncture of the stems and leaves, which are edible before the plant bolts. The blossoms appear cradled by the plant, much like a nurtured child in its mother's arms. Likewise, the Spinach theme generally has enjoyed a healthy, loving childhood where he received the proper emotional tools with which to move forward into adulthood.

These are the very qualities that have prepared him to be an excellent pet owner. His animals will be both children and friends to him, receiving from him the loving nurturance that he received as a child. Even mature Spinach-theme adults will often share games with their pets on the animals' own level. Their joy in their animals will be obvious to all who see them romping together.

Strawberry-Theme Animals: Dignity

The Strawberry theme is a graceful, noble, and dignified animal who handles himself with a sophisticated poise. A quiet pet, he possesses a strong sense of his own beauty, which also touches those around him. Many purebred animals are Strawberry themes. They exhibit a maturity both at rest and at play that is rather extraordinary to watch. One feels in their presence a level of royalty. And although dignity is a quality inherent in all creatures of the earth, the Strawberry theme energizes this characteristic with a special flare.

Even a wild animal with a Strawberry-theme personality will seem to pace his territory as though surveying his domain. And he is doing exactly that. These animals express a wide variety of preferences, based on a certain refinement of their character. They can afford the luxury of turning up their noses at food that does not particularly please them. Although they may seem fussy or finicky at times, they are merely exercising the more refined aspects of their nature. Actually, these pets are quite charming. They are readily trainable and will seem almost embarrassed if they err in a behavior in which they have received training.

Since many people are what we would call Strawberry-deficient—meaning lacking a true sense of their inner beauty and self-worth—Strawberry-theme pets, in their unassuming way, are very worth-affirming animals. Their very presence reflects back to their owners how beautiful and dear their care-takers really are.

Strawberry-Theme Pet Owners: Dignity

Strawberry-theme owners are beautiful, grounded, responsible people. They are earthy, somewhat like Pear themes, but in an elegant manner. Their tastes in clothing, food, and entertainment are refined, and they enjoy being surrounded by beautiful things and uplifting company. It is not uncommon to see them with purebred animals.

Strawberry-themes will lavish both praise and gifts on their fortunate pets. They will treat them to only the best in food, shelter, grooming tools, and toys. "Nothing is too good for my Fluffy," you may hear a Strawberry-theme owner say. The pet of this theme is thus pampered and at times spoiled. He will have his favorite chair or blanket reserved and waiting for him, and basically he is allowed the run of the Strawberry theme's home or property.

Strawberry themes are gracious to their human and animal friends alike, for they are generous people. Dignity being their predominant personality strength, they will see that same beauty and poise in others. They make empowering company for this reason. A Strawberry theme will make you feel not only special but irreplaceably cherished. And don't we all love to be pampered?

Tomato-Theme Animals: Strength, courage

The Tomato-theme pet is noted for his courage. This animal, though instinctually intelligent, is often fearless toward other animals many times his size. Here is the little kitten who will race up and rub noses with a deer. Tomato-theme pets also make excellent guard dogs.

A courageous pet, this theme is a natural rescue animal. Included in the Tomato-theme personality type are seeing-eye dogs, police dogs, and any animals who guard people. Upright posture characterizes the Tomato-theme animal, who seems to welcome life with open arms, paws, or wings. He can face difficulties with great courage. Animals, endowed as they are with sharp senses and keen instincts, all have a bit of the positive Tomato as well as Pear characteristics. Stories abound of pets whose "sixth sense" allows them to foresee imminent violence, threats, and disaster—both man-made and natural—to their owners and themselves.

Perhaps most inspiring of all are the courageous tales of animals who save the lives of complete strangers, sometimes laying down their own lives in the process. Numerous documented cases of animals alerting people to fires, burglaries, earthquakes, and floods focus on pets whose heroism epitomizes the strengthening Tomato-theme animal.

Tomato-Theme Pet Owners: Strength, courage

Tomato-theme owners have tremendous reserves of courage at their disposal. When difficulties present themselves, these brave warriors face them directly, no matter how much energy or stamina is required. Willpower, not to be mistaken with stubbornness or obstinacy, is their battle cry. They do not balk in fearful situations, nor do they back away from obstacles simply because more strength is needed. These are brave, forthright human beings who face their challenges with open minds. Willing to be wrong, they are equally unafraid to be right.

Tomato-theme owners are strong individuals and loving but firm disciplinarians. Their innate bravery, by association with them, breeds fearlessness in their pets. They possess a keen ability to be sensitive to their animal's fears and weaknesses.

Most impressive about the Tomato theme is his ability to love again once a companion animal has died. This individual is not afraid to open his heart to other animals, nor does he fear the pain of future loss. It is said that we draw to ourselves the very thing we most fear—the exact experience we least want to happen. This is not the case with the Tomato theme, who is committed to loving his pets throughout their lifetimes. This owner knows how to grieve when they die, to heal, and then to love again. His animals will be empowered by his gallant approach to pet care.

And when the time arrives for his pet to pass on, this owner, rather than burdening his animal with his own issues, is able to be totally present for his animal friend.

In Conclusion

Many times in my workshops, when we reach the part of the program where we determine theme essences, people will remark to each other at break time, "I am an Orange theme" or "I am a Raspberry theme." This means, respectively, that one *is* the joy or the kindheartedness. More than a few individuals will have tears in their eyes. To identify ourselves with elevating qualities is indeed inspirational. And to view our pets in this same light acknowledges their ability to express the purest qualities in Nature.

A dog who is treated as "just a dog" by his owner will not blossom, much as a plant left untended without proper soil, water, and sunshine may wilt. If the owner were to know, for example, that his dog is an Orange theme, reflecting its quality of pure joy, he might then view his canine companion with higher respect, if not awe.

An animal's mental, emotional, and spiritual needs are equally as important as his physical needs for food and shelter. Our acknowledgment of this principle through the understanding and application of theme essences is a great aid to animals in their evolutionary process, and it is a service they deserve from us as pet owners.

Chapter Summary Outline

1. The term *ego* means identification with our sense of separateness from the Source of life.
2. The personality, an offshoot of the ego, is composed of patterns, habits, likes, and dislikes, with their resulting desires; these desires influence the choices we make in our lives.
3. Animals have "emerging egos," with individualized personalities.
4. Plants do not have individual egos. They do, however, express qualities of nature; these qualities provide the basis for flower essences.
5. The commonly used term *type* remedy refers to a predominant negative quality in an individual's personality.
6. The concept of theme essence, contrarily, identifies people and animals by their predominant and positive personality strengths. For example, a Cherry theme is cheerful, a Lettuce theme is calm.
7. An animal's species or breed, to some extent, will define his theme essence, though individual personality traits may override it.
8. Animals convey their personalities through their behaviors.
9. Give your pet his theme essence when he seems "out of sorts," is fighting an illness, or is simply not acting like himself.
10. Determine your pet's theme essence by watching him rest, play, and interact with others—also ask your children.

11. The theme essence, according to the laws of magnetism (opposites attract and like attracts like as well), may also be determined by what qualities the animal evokes in other pets and people.

12. The theme-essence construct is a valuable tool in helping prospective owners match their personalities with their potential pets.

13. Whereas people commonly have both a theme and a sub-theme (a secondary, slightly less obvious positive quality of their personality), animals often have double themes: two identically strong and positive personality traits.

14. These concepts are generalized. A non-Cherry-theme animal can still be cheerful, and an Avocado theme will possess the strengths of all other theme essences.

15. The theme-essence philosophy may be practically applied to understanding your pet and his needs on deeper levels.

16. This chapter includes profiles of the identifying theme characteristics of the twenty Master's Flower Essences for pets and their owners; it explains the pet's nature and how he will interact with his owner and, respectively, his owner's theme disposition and how he will thus care for his animals.

6

THE PLOT ESSENCE FOR PROBLEMS AND CORRECTIVES

Nature never did betray the heart that loved her.
William Wordsworth

In the previous chapter, we have clarified the use of flower essences to support existing strengths in pets and owners. A particular positive behavior based on an underlying, elevated quality such as kindness or love that is predominant and recurring within the personality is called a theme essence.

Here, we will focus on essence application for specific problems or weaknesses that we want to correct or eliminate, including disturbed behaviors, fears, or any actions troubling to the animal or the pet owner. Most commonly, flower essences are given to fill a need or correct a fault, which is usually expressed through the animal's behavior. This defines the usage of plot essences.

Plot Essences for Animals

Just as an older dog who has consistently acted like a playful puppy all his life would be a Spinach theme, a dog who acts listless, discontented, or "old before his time" *needs* Spinach. This is the definition of the plot application of flower essences.

The word *plot*, borrowed from literary jargon, implies that one must travel from point A to point B to achieve a goal—in the case of Spinach, happiness or peace. Plot application indicates a particular need on the part of the animal; the flower essence acts as a catalyst to restore or awaken the positive quality absent from the pet's personality. By way of example, a skittish animal can benefit from Tomato Essence for strength and courage. The pet who constantly craves attention may be helped with Pineapple Essence for self-assuredness.

Plot essences are divided into two categories: *pivotal* and *peripheral*. Pets—and their owners—will most likely require both kinds of plot essences throughout their lifetimes. Pivotal plot essences apply to life-long and frequently recurring needs, lessons, or challenges, whereas peripheral plot essences are beneficial in specific situations, usually occurring infrequently. Accidents, for example, require peripheral plot essences such as Pear, while ongoing unpleasant or unruly behaviors warrant pivotal plot essences, such as Grape for deep issues of early abandonment.

To repeat: If you suspect anything physically amiss with your pet, a medical evaluation with a qualified veterinarian is advisable. It is important to rule out physical causes for substandard behavior in order to make the best possible essence assessment for your pet. For example, if your cat is suffering from an undiagnosed toothache, administering Corn Essence will not restore his lost energy; once the troublesome tooth is removed—and Pear is given for the extraction trauma—he will most likely experience a surge of energy simply from feeling better.

Another word of caution: Flower essences cannot be used to alter, manipulate, or control an animal's behavior. One woman gave Strawberry to her young cat to correct his clumsiness. Crashing to the floor from high perches on furniture was a behavior disturbing to the pet owner; it remained, evidently, a natural part of the cat's personality. Strawberry Essence, in this case, proved ineffectual because the cat's lack of dexterity was not a problem for him. Perhaps the woman herself would have benefited from an essence—Fig—to help her accept that her cat was simply a bit on the ungraceful side!

Some pets are aloof by nature, especially within the cat family. So, if aloofness is the animal's natural state, this trait will remain unchanged. But if reserve and remoteness are symptomatic of a particular need on the part of your pet, flower essences can initiate profound and visible behavioral improvements.

It is also helpful to understand, as explained in chapter 1, that animals are guided largely by instinct. Thus, telling a cat whose territory is threatened by another cat to "be nice" is missing the boat. This behavior is instinct-based and can be addressed through the gentle use of flower essences such as Grape or possibly Date, for overly expressed territorialism, or Peach, to modify or alleviate the instinctual drive to mark furniture by spraying.

At the same time, the following generalization will apply in most cases: For animals, especially dogs and other more aware species, if the behavior is instinct-based, it may be significantly improved or redirected in positive ways through a flower essence program supplemented with proper training. If the problem is emotion-based, flower essences can help correct the problem. In other words, flower essences will not override instinctive behavior in animals. Essences can, however, help them better adapt to a domesticated existence.

Plot Essences for Pet Owners

Many times, I find in the course of a consultation that the pet owner is as greatly in need of flower essences as the pet—and, to be honest, is often the cause of the problem in the first place. To see the same flower essence needs within a household of people and animals is quite common. Pets and their caregivers share joys and sufferings alike—and their remedies too. In fact, one cannot honestly assess an animal without also considering the owner as part of the picture. If, as it has been said, other people are our mirrors, then pets are our microscopes. Each household contains its own psychological climate, you might say, that is part and parcel of each and every inhabitant.

With explanations of theme essences in the previous chapter and plot essences here, we can begin to understand the subtle relationships between the two concepts. A wonderful match of energies occurs when an owner's theme essence is the same as his pet's plot essence. One will complement the other, energetically speaking. For example, a dog with a Corn theme will be very compatible with an owner whose pivotal plot essence is Corn. In the case of one older woman in need of Corn Essence, she remained very energetic and powerful as long as her dog, himself a vibrant Corn theme, lived with her. He seemed to be her engine to keep things going. After he died, she began to age very quickly. Visits to medical doctors grew frequent; various pains appeared in her joints, and she could no longer walk easily. This had never been a problem while the dog lived, as she had walked him regularly without complaining at all.

One woman, a Peach theme, owned a dog whose pivotal plot essence was also Peach. The dog accompanied the woman everywhere—from room to room, from sofa to chair. When left alone in the house, he would howl loudly and unceasingly until her return. Nothing would pacify him until she reappeared—not the radio, lights left on, or neighbors visiting. When company would stop by, he remained highly demonstrative toward the owner, standing between her and the newcomers until they left the house. We also see how an animal's behavior can be traced back to the way he was previously treated—perhaps in a neglectful home. Thus, an understanding of plot essences and their applications will be of great use to the sensitive pet owner.

The plot-essence section for owners not only shows how they may be in need of essences but how the pet, through his innate sense of commitment and service to his owner, can help his human companions along in their healing process.

With this understanding of plot essences, then, let's review the Master's Essences for plot applications for both pets and their owners. The following definitions encompass pivotal as well as peripheral usage.

Almond Essence for Animals: Self-control

An animal who needs Almond Essence needs it very badly. Almond issues often indicate an animal who is not adjusted to domesticated life. These pets need to learn to balance living in an unnatural environment through moderation in their living habits. Overweight is one symptom; stress is another. Animals limited to small spaces, such as apartments, may be in need of this essence. Indoor cats in particular are accustomed to roaming free in nature; confinement can be a great challenge for them. And living indoors can be more difficult for some breeds than others.

When an animal acts nervous or "cagey"—the equivalent of a person biting his fingernails—Almond is an excellent choice. Also, Almond may assist pets who march repetitively. These pets are simply responding to feeling out of sync with their natural rhythms. This is the essence for pets with nervous habits such as pacing, over-grooming, chewing or gnawing themselves or objects of furniture or clothing, obsessively destroying property, or other frenetic behaviors.

Camile, a black-and-white kitten, exhibited many destructive behaviors that in turn disturbed her owner. She would eat nervously, pull items out of shopping bags, and gnaw on sponges and lamp cords. These excessive and inappropriate behaviors resulted from the loss of her mother while still an infant, requiring that she defend herself. Almond Essence was given, and the owner reported to me, "I almost called you right back. With the first dosage, her pupils widened. Before the essence, she wouldn't look at me directly; she was almost catatonic. She doesn't do that any more, now she confronts me. And she comes when I call her; she never did that before."

Obsessive behaviors indicate one of two things: an issue with the pet or an owner-related problem. Living in an age where stress is oftentimes over-whelming for human beings and destructive to their health on all levels, it is not surprising in the least that they would transmit these imbalances to the pets with whom they intimately share their homes.

Almond Essence for Pet Owners: Self-control

The owner needing Almond Essence is one who is regularly nervous. He may be a chain-smoker or a compulsive eater, or he may exhibit other nervous habits. This essence helps the owner who tends to overwork or overdo his schedule such that he doesn't budget enough quality time to be with his pet. Almond helps him to reprioritize and restore his sense of balance so that there truly are enough hours in the day to get everything done and to have time to spend with his animal friend. Almond gives one a renewed sense of scheduling so that there is always time to "stop and smell the roses."

Animals, who are more in tune with the rhythms of nature, by their very presence can communicate a better sense of how we can use our time more wisely to allow enough time for all activities. This owner can be especially healed by taking regular time out with his pet so that they both can share exercise or other relaxing activities. This individual tends to be high-strung and sometimes scattered; pet companionship will be very nurturing and calming to his nervous system.

The more he tunes in to the quiet nature of his animal—assuming, of course, that the animal is quiet—the more he will find himself relaxing. It is only the owner's state of tension that prevents him from feeling he has enough time to complete necessary tasks.

Almond Essence is superb for owners with problems of living too much through sense stimuli at the expense of their inner calmness. Sexual excess, either in thoughts or actions, is a symptom that calls for this remedy. Also, people who sleep too much, overwork too often, or overextend their energy in any number of ways need Almond Essence. After a while, this lifestyle becomes disturbing to animals, for balance is as essential to their being as it is to their owners. Long walks together in silence will be very calming to their nervous systems.

Apple Essence for Animals: Healthfulness

Apple Essence is strengthening for animals who seem about to become ill or who are recovering from illness. Flower essences, as we have said, do not directly treat physical symptoms, but they do help animals develop a consciousness of health. The false message of illness is that we are weak and vulnerable; Apple Essence, for animals who pick up some form of hypochondria from their owners, can allay these fears. Apple is also a good essence to help create a sense of robustness for the runt of the litter (as is Pineapple).

For pets who have chronic health problems—failing organs, loss of appetite, susceptibility to recurring illness—Apple Essence, along with other supportive measures, can help them adjust to their infirmities.

Sometimes, this essence is called for simply to address bad behavior, as in the case of Minnie. An older cat, mostly feral, Minnie basically kept to herself, hiding under a chair or sofa, except when hissing at other cats or visitors. Again, eliminating possible medical causes for this habit, Apple Essence can help with unhealthy behaviors on the part of the animal.

Apple Essence, especially, is for pets who belong to owners who tend to worry excessively about them, creating an atmosphere of health-related fear and doubt around their ailing companion. Especially when costly treatments or time-consuming procedures are involved, this remedy will be strengthening to an animal. Here we see the dynamic connection between pet and owner. Just as one can reinforce the other with his positive qualities, the opposite can also occur: the owner, usually well-intentioned, may pass on his own fears to his animal. For this reason, it is a good idea for both pet and owner to take Apple Essence at the same time.

Apple Essence for Pet Owners: Healthfulness

Apple essence helps the owner who worries about his pet's health as well as his own. He anticipates problems, as his hypochondria—mild to monumental in severity—includes his animal's well-being and those whom he holds dear. His misplaced care for them tends to backfire, for it draws to him and his pets the very states of illness that he fights so valiantly to avoid. Various health-related fears, doubts, and nagging thoughts of any nature tend to haunt him. He may be prone to over-vaccinating or over-supplementing his pet, silently communicating his own fear to his animal friend.

The owner's fears are easily passed on to his pet, who in return feels vulnerable to illness and depleted by the constant irritation of a worrywart owner. A doubting owner fosters a doubting pet; through questioning his ability to be well, this owner weakens himself with his own thoughts. After a while, such attitudes can be debilitating, even to the healthiest pet. Apple is an important essence in this individual's repertoire of healing therapies, for it cuts to the core of the "doubting Thomas" syndrome.

Apple Essence strengthens one's energy from the level of the spirit through the emotions and mental processes and allows the body a sense of integrated wholeness. It is excellent for recovering from illness, accidents, or surgeries, and preceding them as well, for both pet and owner.

Avocado Essence for Animals: Good memory

Avocado Essence is called for with animals who are unresponsive and dreamy or who seem to be somewhere else in their focus. For any pet who does not respond when called or spoken to, this essence can be very beneficial. Especially since animals by nature live in the moment, it is important to rule out medical causes.

Fluffy's story is a good example of Avocado's application. A stray taken in by a family with a young son, Fluffy tended to remain a roamer. She now responds when her owner calls her for meals and before dark. (This owner also asked playfully if there was an essence for her husband, who has to spend many hours in transit to and from job sites, to encourage him to come home when she calls him!)

Caylin, a six-year-old orange tomcat, responded to Avocado Essence in positive ways noticed by his owner. Previously a bit on the dull side and also a pushover with the other cats, his unresponsive behavior was replaced by a greater alertness and a stronger sense of competition. He had learned, with the aid of this remedy, to stand up for himself.

Avocado Essence may be used for a wide range of behavioral issues, such as for older animals (although you will want to determine whether sight or hearing impairment is a part of the problem), for pets who lose interest in life, and for pets who have lost a human or animal companion and thus express a diminishing sense of their life's purpose.

This is an excellent remedy for animals in training. Its special qualities are focused attention, alertness, and the ability to retain information. It is also used for animals who are being trained when distractions are present, such as other dogs barking, other horses nearby, or children interrupting the lesson. Animals, like people, learn new information at varying speeds with different rates of retention. With respect for individual differences, Avocado Essence can assist the slow learner as well as help to speed results for the more intelligent animals.

Avocado Essence for Pet Owners: *Good memory*

When owners forget the deeper purpose in having pets, they can become neglectful in their pet care, perhaps not spending as much time with their animals as needed. Avocado provides the gentle reminder that owning pets is a privilege. A powerful essence for the owner who forgets routines such as feeding times and their importance for his pet, this essence gets the owner back on track. We could call Avocado a "vibrational training session" for the owner.

On a deeper level, it helps this owner to be mindful of the true purpose of his relationship with his pet and why he befriended the animal in the first place. In this sense, Avocado helps one to remember his priorities and to see the colt in the grown horse, the kitten in the older cat.

It also helps the owner to live more in the moment; a spaced-out owner spaces out the pet. Remember, magnetism is contagious. And since we spread it around whether we are aware of it or not, Avocado encourages us to live more in the present moment, as animals innately do. This essence helps to put us more on their wavelength, enhancing our ability to communicate with them. Avocado Essence may be called "bottled wisdom," for it keeps the owner focused on the special role of pet owner to pet. At its best, an owner strong in this quality is capable of having a profound life-long connection with an animal and, through even one pet, with the entire animal kingdom.

The pet owner strong in Avocado qualities will encourage an animal's natural curiosity and interest in life. Your cat may not be an avid reader, but he will be interested in "reading" you, your house guests, and your new landscaping. An owner who is constantly learning himself will reflect in his pet's innate desire to explore and enjoy new experiences.

On the more mundane level, this essence keeps the owner mindful of the needs of his pet and how to best attend to them. He remembers that the indoor kitten needs regular attention and an energetic playtime, and he is good about changing the litter and bedding. But most of all, he remembers that the essence of any relationship with an animal is based on love, mindfully given.

Banana Essence for Animals: Humility

Banana Essence can work wonders for animals who are overly emotional in their behavior, often for no apparent reason. Emotions and feelings are natural for pets; excessive displays of negative behavior are not. Rocky, a three-year-old neutered male cat, was found by his owner at only a few weeks old. Abandoned and injured, she spent "all day every day" nurturing him back to health. Rocky grew into an unusual cat; he travels with her everywhere, including on camping trips to Yosemite National Park and to fancy hotels for high school reunions. Somehow and somewhere, she confided, he developed a mean streak and would strike out—first at strangers, and then at family and friends. "He simply was into being a brat whenever he wanted, with no warning—totally moody and temperamental."

Although in Rocky's case we could assume that his moods were due to early infancy abandonment issues warranting Grape Essence, in this situation it was Banana that unlocked his truer nature. Now his owner reports, "Wow! Instant sweet kitty!"

For animals who get excessively agitated or upset, Banana offers a calming presence. Animals who are easily spooked can benefit from Tomato Essence; those who seem to get inappropriately riled may find Banana helpful.

Banana Essence is also strengthening for pets who are gentle and sensitive by nature. One needn't consider an essence only for severe behavioral issues; a remedy can be helpful to reinforce positive behaviors as well, as in the case of Leslie, a Gordon setter dog. Leslie was rescued from a shelter the day before he was scheduled to be put to sleep. "There's not an aggressive bone in his body," his owner comments. "He's totally loving; my other dogs dominate him and he's just fine with it." Banana Essence supported his innate sensitivity, according to his owner, who says, "Now he's not as clingy as before. He can sit in the room with the other dogs and doesn't have to push his way past me. Before, he had to be with me all the time."

Banana Essence for Pet Owners: Humility

Banana Essence, which supports humility and calmness, is a tool to help a pet owner see that he may be a part of his pet's problems. "What do you mean I leave Spot alone too often? That dog gets lots of attention!" This is the typically quarrelsome response of a pet owner in need of Banana Essence. Recognizing that he may be in error is the first step in remedying the problem. With the help of Banana Essence, the owner may then be able to place the care for his pet above his own prideful need to be right and self-defensive. Banana reinforces the ability to listen, so the pet owner can admit to making mistakes and can learn from them. If he has treated his pet with less than optimal disciplinary measures or general sensitivity, this essence will help him learn to do so.

Although his role as caregiver to his pet may be great, he may learn to view himself as a means for his animal to have a higher quality of life. People who require this essence need to see the bigger picture—the forest for the trees, so to speak. This is an important essence for owners who are considering relinquishing their pets, basically because they have not been able to "listen to" the animals' needs for clear discipline and regular, loving attention.

These people may be unwilling to admit how much they actually have contributed to their pet's problems, and so, in this sense, it is difficult to acknowledge their need for Banana Essence. The person who can do so by overcoming his own self-protectiveness is on his way to becoming a splendid pet owner, one capable of giving years of quality care to the animals he brings into his household.

Blackberry Essence for Animals: Purity

It may seem that pets exhibiting negative behaviors would need Blackberry Essence in particular. And yet this is often not the case. Date Essence will help to sweeten their actions; Grape Essence assists the pet who behaves badly as a result of lingering abandonment or abuse issues; and Raspberry, diversely, is for the pet who lashes out from a sense of hurt.

Blackberry's placement in an essence program is quite different. Whereas a person is capable of negativity and unkind thoughts, these behaviors are the result of his misuse of will, as described in chapter 1. The faculty of free choice, available to a human being, means that he can choose to move in either positive or negative directions. Animals, basically, do not have that choice. Their decisions are made for them, in a sense, by Nature and are based on survival instincts. Thus, Blackberry Essence does not apply to them as it does to people.

However, this remedy is warranted for the animal whose owner expresses the negative Blackberry state. This pet will tend to absorb his owner's wrong behaviors—and his thoughts as well. Blackberry's key quality is purity of thought—a quality that animals, as a rule, instinctively possess. Usually it is the trials of domesticated life, replete with unhealthy human role models, that cause them to need this remedy.

Lawrence, a four-year-old tomcat, matches this description. His present owner described him as "a bit snobby. If he were human, he would be a crotchety curmudgeon." His previous owner was a woman who had treated him badly and also spoiled him; he had grown accustomed to spending time in the kitchen with the servants. Biting and scratching were Lawrence's common responses if anyone tried to pick him up. His essence program consisted solely of Blackberry. Within a few days, his temperament had changed dramatically for the better.

Blackberry is also an important essence for animals who are no longer able to groom or properly care for themselves. If they seem to have a sense of their own uncleanliness, this essence will help them deal with their physical condition. Jimmy, an eight-year-old German shepherd rescued by his present owner, is incontinent, possibly from a past car accident or abusive treatment. The veterinarian determined that his kidneys had been damaged and recommended an herbal program. After several days of dosing, Blackberry Essence helped with his compulsive habit of self-grooming.

Also excellent for misting in the litter box or places where a pet has soiled or sprayed, Blackberry Essence will help to clean the area. For actual odors or simply "clearing out the energy" in a location, this remedy is useful. And if your pet has been exposed to harmful chemicals, Blackberry, along with medical treatment, is recommended.

Blackberry Essence for Pet Owners: Purity

The pet owner in need of Blackberry essence is one prone to a strain of negativity as infectious as influenza. This unpleasant mental state creates a foul temperament that is distasteful to pets, who tend to withdraw from such an owner as a result. Animals possess a natural telepathy and an ability to read their owners, flawlessly and infallibly. No one, least of all pets who intimately share their owners' environment, likes to be around these carping spirits. Pessimism and downright unkindness repel all who share their space. And what more captive audience is there than housebound animals? Even those pets who live in a yard, pen, or fenced area will be affected by this owner's negative mental state.

When their owner addresses them unkindly in the negative Blackberry state, animals may not understand the meanness of the words, but they unquestionably sense the meanness of spirit behind them. Subjected to verbal cynicism, sarcasm, and the like, animals can exhibit disturbed behaviors. We have received testimonials about cats excreting on rugs, carpets, and bath mats to express their dislike of these attitudes in the people who share their environment.

Blackberry Essence also helps the individual who is working through emotional or psychological issues while seeking clarity and insight. Sensitive and kind by nature, he may feel himself temporarily clouded by difficulties. Blackberry Essence can assist this individual in rehabilitating his emotional awareness.

Cherry Essence for Animals: Cheerfulness

Much as people are prone to moods at times, so are our pets. When they behave in a contrary manner in circumstances to which they normally agree— a trip to the groomers, or a reversal of any behavior in which they have previously been trained and responded—Cherry Essence is recommended. In many ways, pets are like children. They can be ornery at times, grumpy for no apparent reason, or simply bad-tempered (ruling out medical causes). If these negative states are basically transitory in nature, this "sourpuss" behavior indicates the need for Cherry Essence. Cherry trees, by way of a botanical note, are either sweet or sour, much like an animal's temperament. The sweet variety can grow to large heights, whereas the sour kind is much less hearty.

And as mentioned earlier, animals do best with loving guidelines and parameters for what is allowed and acceptable and what is not. If you have trained your dog to not jump on people, then this must remain a non-negotiable house rule.

It is also important for the owner to assess the reason for such moodiness. A cat may not like the new kitty litter and would naturally turn his nose up at it. Or the dog may be unhappy with the new food you are having him sample. Honoring our pets' preferences, within reason, gives them a sense of their place in the household, which is why it is so important to praise them over and over again. However, similar to guiding children, it is important to set consistent boundaries that we are comfortable with as well. A spoiled pet can spoil the entire home; everyone has to live in the same household or property.

Animals may also become moody when they are dealing with difficult situations in their household. They often mirror the moods of their owners.

Also, pets with previously abusive owners may lapse into troubled feelings from time to time. A negative Cherry mood, however, will pass, in contrast to the need for Orange Essence where serious emotional collapse is apparent.

Gabriel, a seven-year-old Australian shepherd, suffered a tragic existence with his previous owner. As a result of earlier mistreatment, he began barking—which resulted in him spending six months outside with a bag of dog food until he was finally given away. He had learned to hide in a corner of his second owner's home. Cherry Essence, for three days in his first program, initiated a noticeable change in his behavior. Cheerier and more friendly to other pets in the household, Gabriel is responding well to this essence.

Cherry Essence for Pet Owners: Cheerfulness

Similar to but not duplicating Blackberry Essence is the grumpy owner in the negative Cherry state of mind. This individual is merely moody, however, and not necessarily aiming his negativity at anyone but himself. This "just plain ornery" state is very upsetting to animals, as it includes an emotional vacillation of mental states that is a bit unnerving to pets who are richly emotional by nature. If a pet is a bit mopish, it behooves the owner to see if his animal is mirroring his own mood. Animals thrive in an emotionally balanced household and immediately sense when any one of its members is unhappy or gloomy.

A "yo-yo" owner can learn even-mindedness from his animals, as they can teach him Nature's lesson of good cheer. It is important for our own health to play with our pets, even to sing and dance with them—basically, to not let life's endless annoyances cloud our happiness. The next time you feel grumpy, try dancing with your bird on your shoulder, teaching your dog a new song, or inventing a dance to share with your cat. Watch what it does for both of you!

This owner is also one who is prone to use inconsistent discipline with his pets. While he may think that he is treating them well by occasionally allowing them to break the established rules, he is actually doing them a great disservice, as irregular training confuses animals. They may even look up (or down) at him with an expression that may be translated as, "Huh? But it was OK to do this last time!"

Cherry Essence helps this owner to be more even-minded with his animals and to reach a level of detachment in his disciplinary methods so that he can feel comfortable with the rules he imposes instead of feeling apologetic or tyrannical.

And for the passing of a companion animal, Cherry Essence can help the owner to stabilize the natural flood of emotions. One owner, dealing with the death of her ten-year-old cat, reported, "At one point, I felt that I was crying too hard for comfort. I took a few drops of Cherry and the crying stopped. It has been almost three months since he died and I can talk of him and look at photos of him without feeling depressed or too sad. In fact, I smile whenever I think of him."

Coconut Essence for Animals: Upliftment

Coconut Essence is very powerful for animals. It supports their innate desire to evolve. Symptomatically, this translates as a certain uneasiness in their domesticated environment or bodily condition.

Coconut is good for behavior reflecting chronic pain, such as arthritis or healing from an accident. And while this essence will not treat the pain itself, it can effect a positive change in the animal's behavior. Pear is helpful as well, but considering the different way that animals experience pain, Coconut helps them with another aspect: how to deal with it in ways that make them more comfortable with their situation.

Daisy, a twelve-year-old, seventy-pound, Samoyed–yellow Lab mix has suffered from a shaky, arthritic back left leg. She would often groan and freeze up as though the uncomfortable leg had tired her and caused a great deal of pain. Now, according to her owner, she's perkier. Thus, Coconut Essence is good for older animals who get "creaky" in their limbs. It doesn't take a veterinarian to see when an animal walks with pained joints. Difficulty climbing up or down stairs, slowness in moving out of a sleeping position, and a visible way of favoring certain body parts to avoid strain on other areas are all signals for Coconut.

For some animals, a feeling of "I can't" will block their abilities to shine as show animals. Royalty, a nine-year-old show horse, was described as being well-built, versatile, and a horse who "couldn't stand up for himself."

His essence program included Coconut to help him transcend the sense of limitation of his own capabilities. These attitudes are often owner-induced but nonetheless supremely reversible.

Also, for the pet who loses a companion through death or other separation, Coconut Essence is recommended as an adjunct to Grape.

Coconut Essence for Pet Owners: Upliftment

Coconut Essence is for the pet owner who gives up on his pet. At the end of his rope with their recurring inconveniences, he is ready to throw in the towel and see them on their way. People who abandon their animals or take them to rescue facilities seriously need this essence. It is the "commitment essence." Coconut helps to restore a sense of perseverance and, even more importantly, the recognition that there is a perfect answer to every pet problem.

Rather than giving up—and giving up on—the pet, this essence helps the owner to see what he needs to learn from the situation. Sometimes, the lesson is to "look before you leap" and not bring home another precious little kitten who will grow into an adult cat with ongoing needs for nutritious food and active companionship. When pets begin to feel like a problem, it is time for the "solution essence": Coconut.

Coconut Essence (as well as Grape) is also recommended for the pet owner who loses a pet or, in fact, for the owner of aged animals who will be passing on soon. It allows us to focus on the beautiful lessons we can learn from them as they leave us and also to turn our thoughts to the many ways they have taught and inspired us during their years in our care. The more we can express the priceless lesson of Coconut, the more supportive we can be to our animal friends at the time of their passing.

Corn Essence for Animals: Vitality

Corn Essence helps to restore a sense of adventure and play to pets who are relocated or taken to a new home. During the adjustment phase when everything is foreign to them, they may instinctively withdraw until they become familiar with the new location, sounds, smells, sights, and especially the presence of other animals. Corn Essence helps them integrate into a new environment with a burst of energy to explore, investigate, and once more to enjoy.

Cats, who are particularly environment-oriented, do well with this remedy during times of change in their environment. Sometimes even rearranging the furniture can be somewhat upsetting to felines; this essence helps them work with these changes in positive ways.

Corn Essence does not supply physical vitality as do vitamins and nutritious foods but rather a renewed interest in life. It can also spark an animal's curiosity in what is going on around him—outside the window or house, in the field, and so on. Corn awakens a pet's natural zest for new experiences. For this reason, it is important that he have safe access to the outdoors, especially in urban settings.

Ruling out medical causes, animals too can be couch potatoes. Especially if the owner tends toward sluggishness, this essence can help both pet and owner to find inspirational ways to use their time together.

Older animals who have lost some of their spunkiness due to the normal aging process rather than a specific illness or infirmity will act perkier and peppier on Corn Essence. Rags, a twelve-year-old mixed-breed canine, responded well to this remedy. A regular employee of his owners' business, he literally "hopped around the office—people were asking what he was on," the staff reported.

Pets who for various reasons have had their energy exhausted may also respond well to Corn Essence.

Corn Essence for Pet Owners: Vitality

A boring owner makes for a boring pet, says one dog trainer who has seen many lackluster individuals bring their lifeless animals to her for training. Express your enthusiasm to your canines, she recommends. Lavish non-subtle praise on them for learning their commands. Share their excitement, and let them share yours.

Some individuals who bring pets into their homes, even if not old in years, harbor old attitudes; they may be inactive, listless, or just can't seem to "jump-start" themselves.

Corn Essence, "the energizer," abounds with enthusiasm and joy. The owner who procrastinates could be building new pens for his pets. The sofa slouch, nursing a bulging potbelly, could be out jogging with his llama.

Animals inherently love to express themselves through movement and will undoubtedly love their owner's company on their romps. Exercise, the experts say, is the best cure for lethargy as well as depression. Try sharing an "endorphin treat" with your animal friend. Run, jump, prance, and play. Corn Essence creates a win-win situation between owners and their pets; everyone feels better through productive activity shared with interspecies friends.

A move to a new home, beginning a new job, starting a new school term: all are perfect times for Corn Essence. Energy begets more energy; joy multiplies into more joy. Your pets will reflect these changes in you—and quickly, too. Your enthusiasm for life will create an environment for an animal with a heightened interest in life.

Date Essence for Animals: Sweetness, tenderness

As mentioned with Cherry Essence, sometimes animals can be just plain ornery. When their feistiness carries a certain edge to it, Date Essence can be helpful. Just as people can have their "off" days, so can pets. And they express it much as we do—by being crabby, picky, and downright irritable.

Although animals are not capable of expressing criticism and judgment as human beings do, they can still convey their dislikes and disfavor with their surroundings and those sharing it. Pets in the negative Date condition tend to pick on other animals. In fact, the need for this essence is most easily noticed in households with more than one pet. If you see one pet picking on another, similar to the negative Grape state's bullying behavior, it is highly recommended that this essence be given. And since animals respond so quickly to flower essences, much relief will be afforded to the animal who is being picked on.

The behavior of one dog sweetened considerably on Date Essence. A black Lab–Irish setter mix was previously described as touchy and jealous by his owner. After having the Date Essence rubbed into his coat, he is now "really sweet to other dogs. He licks their ears. He's still a bit touchy, but nothing like before the remedy," his owner said.

Date Essence for Pet Owners: Sweetness, tenderness

An owner lacking Date's sweetness is sour indeed. This owner needs help, and quickly. Those in the negative Date condition are unwelcoming and inhospitable; they breed unfriendly and unmagnetic attitudes through being judgmental, thereby creating an invisible wall of separation around themselves.

It is one thing to discriminate but quite another to judge. These owners need to learn Date's lesson of accepting everyone as a part of their family. Pets of these owners, understandably, become irritable and irritating. If multiple pets share the household, they may all pick up on the owners' lack of charity. This tends to be a home with lots of fighting, squabbling, hissing, and growling. The pets will be defining strong territorial boundaries—"this is my bed" or "that is my sofa to lounge on"—and anyone who oversteps these definitions is asking for a tussle or a swat with the paw.

The owner strong in this quality, on the other hand, will find his pets reflecting his hospitality. They will be the first ones at the door to greet guests. Their sweet-natured temperaments will extend to their expressed caring for other pets in the household or barnyard in an almost protective manner. You may find them grooming each other or even napping in each other's arms. Their loving gestures will melt an owner's heart.

Fig Essence for Animals: Flexibility

Some animals, through wrong training, get the message that they are somehow not OK, that some part of their behavior is not acceptable to the owner. As the animal places high value on this relationship, anything that mars its placidity can create a sense that something is wrong with him. It is for this reason that pets should neither be yelled at nor spoken harshly to. Firmness is one thing; meanness is another. Thus, Fig is one of several essences needed by a pet whose problems are often owner-related.

Many animal species are highly trainable and respond beautifully to consistent, firm, and loving discipline. Any mixed messages from their owners, however, create deep confusion for pets. It is these animals who can benefit from Fig Essence. And if you acquire an animal whose past history is unavailable, it is wise to give him Fig Essence at some point during your care for him.

Herbert, a black-and-white tomcat presently living in his second home, was put on a program that included Fig Essence. He always seemed on his guard and would not let his new owner anywhere near him. Previously belonging to a woman who had yelled at him, he grew confused with so many rules; he was no longer certain what behavior was acceptable and what was not allowed. Adapting to one restriction after another, Herbert became an animal who could not seem to figure out what to eat or, in fact, what was expected of him. He responded beautifully and immediately to a Fig Essence program, according to his owner, and now seems to "fit in with the other animals in the house."

For fussy pets who do not tolerate food even when enough variety is offered, or for animals who seem whiny or somehow discontent under the most pleasant circumstances, Fig can help them adjust and enjoy the services rendered them by an accommodating owner.

This remedy is also advised in conjunction with Avocado Essence for training animals. In learning new rules, it is helpful to have a certain flexibility and thus receptivity to changing old patterns—a particular strength of Fig Essence. Also, for breaking existing bad habits, these two essences are recommended. For any variations in eating or sleeping habits, alterations in established routines, or any changes in the home or its residents that affect the pet's lifestyle, Fig is a wonderful adjunct.

Fig Essence for Pet Owners: Flexibility

The owner in the negative Fig state is rigid by nature. His basic discomfort in accepting himself as he is creates uncomfortable animals. Somehow, nothing is ever quite right for him. There may be lots of crying, scurrying, or whining by pets in this house. He is constantly correcting and overdisciplining his animals in an attempt to get his own life in better order.

Although this household may be fastidiously organized, it will lack a certain easygoing flow. An unending series of rules are created in an attempt at a togetherness that never quite happens. Rather than arranging the home for the animals, it is they who are expected to conform to the owner's rules: "Stay away from the china cabinet"; "Leave the houseplants alone"; "Don't track mud on the linoleum." And these kinds of rules are invariably broken by pets in training. In the home of the negative Fig owner, no one can relax.

An owner who learns the lesson of Fig will raise self-accepting, confident pets who recognize themselves as respected members of the household. Any tension-based health problems may begin to remedy themselves at this point. Pets who are jittery will be able to calm down. Animals who seem slightly on edge will relax. Their body language will soften, and you will see comfortable, happy pets.

Grape Essence for Animals: Love, devotion

Grape is an excellent "all-purpose" essence to have on hand for your pet's range of behavioral changes reflective of some aspect of neediness—abandonment, jealousy, whining, loneliness, clinginess, or its opposite, aloofness. The essence for pets who are left virtually forgotten by their owners—caged, penned, leashed, or corralled—is Grape.

Perhaps he is reacting to new, difficult, or unpleasant circumstances. Consider, for example, the meticulously clean twelve-year-old house cat who began defecating in every room of his owner's home when the woman's new boyfriend began visiting on a regular basis. Whether the cat exhibited jealousy, demand for attention, or disapproval of the woman's chosen partner, his behavior highlighted a problem begging for a solution, clearly indicating the need for Grape Essence.

For the blending of households when your cat is no longer "top dog" and loses interest in food, for withdrawn or bullying behavior when other pets are brought into the home, and for the animal who whines or cries for no apparent reason, Grape is highly recommended. Also for those pets who behave in an overly or inappropriately territorial manner, this essence calms them almost immediately.

In addition, the severing of ties due to children in the household moving out or the divorce of their caretakers oftentimes cause behavioral disturbances in animals. Grape also helps a pet who becomes listless after the passing of another pet or person in the household, especially if they had been close companions for some time. For the grief of animal mothers when their babies are given away, this essence (in close proximity to Peach) in her water and rubbed behind her ears offers special comfort.

Grape essence is also useful for the lonely pet or, conversely, "the loner." Animals who are repeatedly left alone for long periods without the company of people or other animals may develop behavioral problems. "I can guard against thieves, I can guard against pests," says a dog in a cartoon strip, chained on a leash in an empty field. "But how do you guard against loneliness?"

One house cat whose owner traveled frequently had developed a loud, mournful, yelping cry during her owner's absence. The cat would walk into a room and, for no apparent reason, cry as though she were being strangled. After three days with Grape added to her drinking water, the crying stopped completely. Had the essence also been applied topically, results might have been noticed even sooner.

Pets who are overly clingy rather than merely affectionate can exhibit remarkable responses to Grape. (Peach Essence is also recommended.) For the cat who monopolizes a lap though set aside many times or for the dog who won't let you out of his sight even for a moment, this essence is well worth trying. One little dog, rescued from an animal shelter, had grown accustomed to following his owners around from room to room. A few days on Grape found him behaving in a more relaxed manner—no longer pacing and following nervously, no more yelping, and now wagging his tail often.

In the case of Rory, we see how Grape allowed an otherwise standoffish cat the freedom to enjoy the indoors and the company of others in the household rather than being limited by an adaptive behavior in which she had learned to keep to herself in a family of many other pets. Rory, "the aloof one," as her owners call her, was the only one who kept her distance from me when I went to consult with a family who owned six cats, even though feeding time had arrived. "Unapproachable by nature" describes Rory. This independent loner had always slept outdoors in the nearby fields, playing with the resident foxes in her youth. If left alone with the two manx cats whom she had mothered, Rory routinely picked fights with them. Following only two days on Grape, she began sleeping indoors on the bed. "This has never happened since we moved into this house three years ago," I was told by an incredulous owner. "Rory wouldn't even come into the house before. We thought she just didn't need anything from us. Her behavior now is unbelievable."

For animals who are bad-tempered or even potentially dangerous, Grape is recommended. Jasmine, a beautiful green-eyed, white-haired cat whose owner had nicknamed her "the cat from hell," apparently had "an attitude." Described as mean-spirited with a nasty disposition, fourteen-year-old Jasmine had been severely torn apart by a dog in her youth, which, according to her owner, had rendered her unpleasant company ever since. He reported, "She's nice when she drinks her Grape water. She even goes outside now, for the first time in two years." And for animals who are ill-tempered for no apparent reason, Grape is also indicated.

When new pets are brought into the household, behaviors such as possessiveness and jealousy are quite common (see "Dominance, Hierarchy, and Territory" in chapter 3). Friday, an older black cat, began swatting at the new feral kitten who had been moved into her home. When dosed with Grape Essence, Friday began grooming him instead. This behavior does not occur often, I was told, but does repeat itself. Grape, when reapplied, invariably initiates the same affectionate and demonstrative response in Friday each time this negative pattern reappears.

For the boarding of a pet whose behavior is problematic stemming from abandonment and loneliness rather than the shock of the move (which would indicate the need for Pear Essence), Grape is recommended. If both issues are present, Grape and Pear may be administered, though in close proximity rather than in combination—Grape one day followed by Pear the next.

Any change or disruption in environment or routine may cause behavioral imbalances in your pet, which can be dramatically remedied by flower essences. Pear Essence is most helpful in emergencies, whereas Grape is useful when people or other animals in your pet's environment are involved.

For a pet's loss of an owner or other animal friend, as explained more fully in chapter 7, Grape is the essence for bereavement and grieving. When animals are raised together and spend their entire lifetimes in each other's company, one will inevitably die before the other. Grape Essence helps the remaining pet to cope, to grieve, and to heal.

Grape Essence for Pet Owners: Love, devotion

As the owner in the negative Grape state has many expressions, a variety of negative behaviors will be reflected in the home of this owner. Least difficult of all is the lonely owner. If he can transmute his sense of isolation, he and his pets will be able to share a deeply fulfilling relationship. Otherwise, he will merely translate his sense of bereftness to them, fostering lonely animals. Grape Essence is also imperative for the owner who leaves his pets alone too often without realizing the impact it has on them.

If the owner is cruel, his household companions will receive the brunt of his meanness. Even a sharpness in the owner's voice indicates his need for Grape Essence. Abuse sometimes happens to people as well as to animals. This remedy also addresses any abuse that has transpired in the owner's life.

But more often than not, the Grape-deprived owner is simply one who feels somehow incomplete and lacking love in his life. Perhaps a spouse has died. The owner may have moved to a new location due to a job transfer and not yet established a circle of friends. Or perhaps he is one of many who suffer from the cultural loneliness inherent in a mobile, overworked society.

Condolence cards for pets and entire books on pet bereavement suggest how dearly owners care for their pets and also that pet loss is a widespread experience. Animals live shorter lives and thus pass in and out of ours on a somewhat regular basis. Grape Essence can help the owner deal with this time of transition.

This individual, through the assistance of Grape Essence and a commitment to changing his attitudes, can become a very deeply loving pet owner. By giving the love to his animal that he wishes to receive, he will find his sense of loneliness and neediness dissipating. This state of emotional bankruptcy may be transformed instead into deeply loving bonds with animals who can then literally blossom under his loving care; his pets will express a certain fullness. Receiving regular doses of love will reflect in the pets' glowing coats and radiantly focused eyes. A loved animal is a loving animal.

Lettuce Essence for Animals: Calmness

Younger animals of any breed and species, much like children, are often restless. Their attention spans may last several seconds to a few minutes.

Lettuce Essence is a gently focusing essence that allows animals to calm down. Cork, a two-year-old rat terrier, relaxed considerably on Lettuce Essence—even though he nearly caused his owner to spill the bottle out of excitement as she was applying his dosage!

Analysis of the lettuce plant itself has revealed minute amounts of a chemical known for its hallucinogenic properties. Although no physical trace of the chemical makes its way into the essence, we often, if not always, see threads of similarities from seed to plant to food source to blossom and back to seed. Lettuce follows this pattern.

Lettuce will not take the spirit out of an animal; it will merely help to remove the distractions around truly calm energy. Bogie, a two-year-old pug, is a regular attendant at one of my Los Angeles lectures periodically conducted in his owners' dining room. Bogie loves to bounce around during the class. And although he does not care for the brandy-preservative taste of the essence, he responds nonetheless. Within ten minutes of having a few drops rubbed on his gums and into his coat, he can be found sleeping on the nearest lap. Lettuce Essence, then, helps to remove the tension from an animal's sheer joy in physical play and exercise without altering or compromising his natural personality.

If guests come to visit an animal's household, Lettuce Essence will help him to not become agitated by new people in his territory. Sometimes animals simply "go nuts" when guests arrive. Humans each have a unique smell, sound, and appearance with which the pet will need to familiarize himself. Lettuce, then, helps pets who are already wound up as well as older animals who need to accommodate new energies in their existing environments.

For quiet-natured animals who seem to be more withdrawn than calm, Lettuce Essence is suggested. Domino, a Siamese cat who used to jump two stories down from his previous owner's apartment to maintain his distance, is a case in point. Miss Fetacina, a longhaired tabby in the same household, also exhibited a need for this remedy. Remaining aloof from the other cats, she responded well to an essence program that included Lettuce.

Both Lettuce and Almond Essences address the quality of calmness. Almond is called for when the animal's behavior contains an obsessive, compulsive, or nervous element; Lettuce relates more to a restless energy, at times emotionally based. Thus, for animals who are angry, Lettuce is suggested. If the anger is based on an identifiable source of hurt, you might also try Raspberry Essence.

Lettuce Essence for Pet Owners: Calmness

The owner lacking the calmness of Lettuce may be given to emotional upheaval. Here too is the owner in need of more patience in caring for his pets. His tension is easily transmitted to his pets, who are themselves always a bit edgy. Those in his presence are somewhat likely to become jittery, overexcited, and thus uncomfortable—especially his animals.

He may also have trouble expressing himself—being unable to share his feelings and communicate what he needs to say to people—or he may simply lack the concentration to put his thoughts clearly into words. This "static in the attic" atmosphere can be unnerving to pets, who thrive on calming stability. People who are prone to angry outbursts can benefit from this essence. A remedy assisting with communication skills, Lettuce Essence helps people to not speak out in anger, which they usually regret doing once their emotions have calmed.

Especially for sensitive animals in the household, strongly expressed emotions and loud voices can be disturbing to their physical and emotional health. Lettuce Essence for the owner can allow everyone in the household to relax. Pets who are both sensitive and strong enough can be a great source of comfort to their human friends. Once Lettuce begins to take effect, the entire household will seem more quiet and soft.

Orange Essence for Animals: Joy

As mentioned in chapter 4, pets become unhappy or depressed for blatantly predictable reasons: abandonment, abuse, or neglect. And the loss of a human or animal companion due to death or relocation calls for Orange Essence as well, often in addition to Grape Essence. Also depressing for them is having to adapt to indoor life, cages, yards, fenced pens, or other unnatural situations. Consequently, animals can often become listless, despairing, or physically ill. Studies have shown that depression weakens the immune system, which means that any propensity toward illness will be magnified.

Pets who live with depressed owners pick up some measure of their sadness. Oftentimes, the animal will try to help the owner out of his depression, usually with excellent results. For ongoing illness or despair—or any situation with a lot of emotional heaviness—Orange Essence is recommended. Also, pets with a history of multiple homes can be helped by this essence.

Animals who have been declawed, debarked, or otherwise altered in ways that are highly unnatural to their wild state (excluding surgeries such as spaying and neutering that reduce a critical overpopulation problem) will benefit from this essence. In her prime, Taylor had been a show dog. Then debarked and locked in a garage for over a year, she later developed massive tumors and a leaky bladder. Her present owner gave her a program of Orange Essence, to which she responded in a matter of days, even though physical symptoms persisted.

In addition, physical restriction, resulting from an impaired ability to move, is depressing to animals. This remedy assists animals who through injury, age, or illness have lost the ability to walk, run, fly, or otherwise freely use their bodies.

Pets as well as people can suffer from hormonally-based depression. And whereas flower essences do not work on the level of physical imbalance, they can address the issues around or behind the upheaval of hormone-induced mood swings. During pregnancy or after birth are routinely positive times to administer Orange Essence.

Animals who are grieving the loss of other animal friends or humans will be comforted by this essence. Grape, too, is recommended, though in close proximity rather than at the same time. Grieving is natural when a loved one leaves, as expressed in chapter 3 by Lilly and Freckles, the rabbits whose family were killed by a rattlesnake.

Orange is recommended for any kind of setback—for animals battling terminal illness or any recurrence or relapse of debilitating illness, for animals who have been exhausted or otherwise pushed past their limits, for animals who seem to have lost their spirit, and for pets after particularly long birthings. These situations, although similar to the need for Corn

Essence, all possess an element of suffering, whereas Corn Essence is more for issues of sluggishness or laziness. Basically, any issue that includes an element of emotional struggle may respond to Orange Essence.

Orange Essence for Pet Owners: Joy

The home of an Orange-deficient owner will be perceived by its animal inhabitants as heavy. There's no joy, no hope—people may drag their feet, and pets will tend to drag their paws. Sometimes an owner may be going through serious clinical depression, which places all the animals in the household in a "flighty" position, as though, if given the chance, they'd rather run away. In part, their reaction stems from an innate recognition that despair is completely foreign to our true nature in joy. To live otherwise is unnatural to them, and coping can be very difficult.

Animals can be wonderful sources of support during times of Orange depression. They can entertain and amuse, reminding their owners in little ways of life's innate joy. Sometimes all it takes is a romp with the dog or a song with the parrot to help the owner begin to transmute his sorry state of despair.

In consideration of his animals, the owner in a state of depression needs to address his problems and uproot them as quickly and thoroughly as possible. "You can lead a horse to water," the saying goes, "but you can't make him drink." This owner needs to help himself and drink deeply of the water of joy, ending his joy-draught for both the sake of his animals and himself.

There is no faking it with animals, who sense our innermost feelings perhaps more clearly than we ourselves do. Through getting involved with other people and shifting our focus to volunteer groups or special projects with family or friends, we can lighten our own minds and provide our pets with a happier emotional climate.

Peach Essence for Animals: Selflessness

Peach Essence is for the pet who is overly demonstrative toward his owner. Following the owner from room to room, or fence to fence if outside, this animal is typically clingy. The cat who refuses to leave your lap under any circumstance falls into this category. Often, animals who were weaned too early exhibit this type of behavior, which can be lessened or eliminated with Peach Essence. Grape, for abandonment and neediness, can nicely supplement Peach for these same issues.

Other related pet behaviors correctable with Peach Essence are drooling, kneading with their claws as though nursing, and attempted suckling on older animals of their own or other species or on people. They may also tend to bite or chew on your clothing, furniture, or household items. These behaviors are completely reversible with conscientious flower essence care, though several months on essences may be necessary to correct this problem.

Animals who are removed from their natural habitats do become dependent on us to meet their physical needs, but those who are unable to remain *emotionally* independent can benefit from Peach Essence.

Peach Essence is basically for overpossessive animals—for demanding pets who don't seem to "get it" when you feel that you need more space or privacy, for pets who follow you around, and for animals who cannot seem to let go of a previous owner or a child leaving home. Animals who demand our energy, insist on meals before feeding time, or display excessive territorialism will benefit from this essence.

Also, for animals who do not get along well with other pets in the household or on the property, Peach Essence offers a more expansive, embracing quality to their personalities. Robert, a white and gray moustached tomcat whom his owner described as acting more like a dog than a cat, had difficulty integrating with other pets in the household until being given a program that included Peach Essence. Now he is no longer "bent out of shape and upset by one other cat in particular," his owner observed.

This remedy is valuable for the mother whose babies are being given away. Even when the separation is temporary—for example, when the young are taken to the veterinarian—her distress may be soothed with Peach Essence. Without anthropomorphizing, loss of one's young is a devastating experience. Granted, this is far less the case in an ant colony than for a mother whose child is going off to college. In these circumstances, it is a good idea to also give Orange Essence in close proximity to Peach.

When younger animals are brought into a household with other pets of seniority, the older residents may need Peach Essence to help them relax their territorial instincts. A giant leap in awareness is needed for a pet to accept another animal into his domain. Grape Essence for jealousy and feeling threatened is also useful in this situation.

Peach Essence for Pet Owners: Selflessness

Peach is another essence in which the owner's need for this remedy is transmitted to his animal companions, causing problems for them. Codependent relationships between people and their pets do exist. Peach-deficient, conditional love creates a relationship based on the owner wanting his pet to fill his emotional needs rather than sharing his joy with his animal friend. When we depend on another being for our sense of wholeness, the fear always lurks that whatever is filling our needs may desert us and that we will be left empty and alone once more. This fear, indicating the need for Peach Essence, tends to create a constant tension within the owner and an inability to enjoy the gift of our animal friendships. Here we see the overprotective owner, the fretting pet guardian, the individual whose fear seriously undermines his ability to freely love his animals.

Peach Essence helps the owner understand this basic truth: The more we give, the more we receive. The owner who smothers instead of mothers; who places demands on his pets; who loves with "strings attached," usually requiring certain behavior from the animal—these are the owners in need of Peach Essence.

The animal caregiver who will benefit from this essence is one who needs to learn a healthy balance between care and overconcern for his animals. Animals in a positive-Peach household receive back the freely given love that they bestow on their guardians. This remedy can also assist the owner who seems to not care enough for his pets, putting other less important issues before their well-being. Also, people who lose a pet by death or other separation and adopt a new animal with the express purpose of replacing the departed one can be helped by Peach Essence. All too easily, they may unconsciously place unrealistic expectations on the newer animal to behave like the older one.

Pear Essence for Animals: Peacefulness

Pear Essence helps restore peace to a distraught, disturbed, or injured animal. Thus it is the essence of choice in emergencies and a must for your first-aid kit. If you must board your puppy during a vacation, new people and foreign environments indicate the need for Pear. This essence is excellent for calming a pacing horse. And for any animal whose pregnancy is nearing term, throughout labor, and several days afterward, Pear provides noticeable benefits. We have received more testimonials from pet owners over the years about Pear than any other essence.

Pets, like people, thrive on regularity, security, and stability. Add these conditions to their lives, along with Pear Essence for upsets and accidents, and they may spend many fruitful years with you. Animals can suffer immensely when the familiar and comfortable are removed from their routines. Any break in an animal's familiar schedule, large or small, can cause him anxiety. Anything from moving to a new location to a change in feeding cycles can be disturbing and stressful to them. Thus a consistent schedule contributes to optimum well-being, which is apparent through sleek coats, healthy gums and teeth, strong bones, shining eyes, and a natural interest and curiosity in their environment.

It is quite common for panic, treatable with Pear, to accompany a livestock ranch's yearly roundup. Amidst a climate of general chaos and disorientation, the calves are separated from their mothers for the routine cattle branding, dehorning, and castration. Last spring, a woman visiting a ranch during roundup time "just happened" to be carrying a bottle of Pear in her pocket. She poured the remedy into the calves' watering troughs. Within one hour—longer than usual for results, since not all the calves drank immediately—she observed that they had all settled down. Her comments: "This is completely unusual; I have never witnessed this calming before." Normally, the calves would remain restless and inconsolable until the procedure was completed.

Injured pets who must be left overnight at an animal hospital, separated from their owners and subjected to the sight, sound, and smell of foreign animals, may find comfort in Pear Essence. Also, after surgery, as well as several days before, is an excellent time for Pear, as Thomas's story illustrates.

When only a year old, this little poodle was attacked and severely bitten by a larger farm dog. Nearly dying on the operating table had caused additional shock and trauma to his body. Upon returning home, Thomas remained listless and practically unmoving. Twenty-four hours after being placed on Pear, he resumed eating and drinking as well as playing—a recovery time cut in half. Now in excellent health and spirits, this spunky little dog is five years of age.

If your pet becomes ill, Pear provides a calming effect and thus allows other medications or therapies to work more effectively. One woman reported dramatic Pear results for her tabby. The cat had experienced severe muscle spasms following a cycle of antibiotics for cystitis. "Many times that night, we thought she would go," the woman explained. "Pear brought her out of the spasms and calmed her down almost instantly." In this case, Pear prevented further upset from the disturbing symptoms.

Six-year-old Tramps, a mixed breed of dog, received relief from Pear after a stomach tumor had left him lethargic—neither eating, drinking, nor evacuating. His gums had turned white, and he could only drink water through a turkey baster. A worried owner interpreted Tramps's walking-off-into-the-woods behavior to mean that his time was near. "Since putting him on Pear," he reported, "he's gone from not being able to move to sitting up. Before Pear, he was breathing so shallowly that we thought he had died." Some days later, I heard that Tramps was back to his old self—eating, drinking, and eliminating as usual. Although still unable to stand, he could at least manage to roll over.

Often animals suffer without showing it. One reason they adapt to, or hide, their pain so well is purely instinctual—to expose weakness in the wild virtually guarantees attack by predators. Pear may be administered to an animal whether it is conscious or unconscious. Many pet owners carry this remedy with them in case of emergency. Panic, anxiety, and disorientation are commonly treatable symptoms in a crisis where time may be of the essence. As mentioned earlier, Pear also nicely supplements medical care for your pet without causing conflict or contraindications. Do be sure, however, to choose a method of application which will neither alarm nor disturb your pet—a light misting, for instance, versus rubbing the essence into his gums, which may be too invasive for a traumatized animal and dangerous for you.

How to treat the common behavioral problem of biting? Fish, a sleek black nine-year-old house cat, responded almost instantly to Pear Essence. "She goes on overdrive," her owner had observed over the years. "She bites when she's overstimulated, mad, or frustrated. I suspect bad weaning is partly responsible. Also, she was queen of the house until I brought in other cats." Since biting, in her case, was attributed to conflict—disturbance of routine as a kitten (improper weaning), displacement in the household (other pets brought into the picture), and moving to a new house—Fish was given Pear Essence. (Had the biting been a fear-based reaction, I would suggest Tomato; had it been a weaning issue alone, Peach; and for jealousy, feeling left out, or vying for attention, Grape.) Thus, Fish provides us with a prime example of the basic precept of flower essences: Treat the personality and not the symptoms; address the individual and not the disease.

Animal trainers, breeders, veterinarians, and herbalists report using Pear Essence with many cats, dogs, and other animals. They find that results are powerful and immediate. As a first-aid remedy, Pear is useful both indoors and outside for scrapes, bruises, falls, bites, stings, and burns. Pear is restorative and calming to both wild and domestic animals.

And if it is your pet's time to die, Pear Essence, the "rest in peace" remedy, can help calm him at the time of his passing. (Information on bereavement for a pet's passing can be found in chapter 7.)

Pear Essence for Pet Owners: Peacefulness

Pear is indicated for a pet owner in times of trauma. For accidents, illness, and surgeries, this remedy may be of great assistance. Also, when an owner is in crisis brought on by his pet's injuries, Pear Essence can calm everyone intimately involved. We are more helpful to our injured animal with our own peace of mind restored and operative. Thus, Pear is an excellent essence for pets and their owners to take at the same time. And remember, one needn't be a total "basket case" to benefit from Pear. Even feeling a bit off balance or out of sorts is enough reason to take this important remedy.

For owners who are quarrelsome, anxious, disturbed in some way, or antagonistic to others, Pear Essence offers a sense of peacefulness. When people have to face difficult situations that cause them distress, this herbal tincture can be greatly pacifying. For some people, visiting relatives can be traumatic; for others, asking for a raise at the office is upsetting. Whatever the cause, the effect is the same: loss of peace of mind.

Even a stressful day of running errands can indicate a need for Pear Essence. Anything that negatively influences us, either physically or emotionally, can cause further upset if the process is not halted. With peace restored, problems cease to exist—in our minds, if not outwardly.

Pineapple Essence for Animals: Self-assuredness

Pineapple Essence assists pets who are insecure and need a stronger sense of their own identity and placement in a household, especially where children or other animals are involved. An animal's sense of smell is many times more acute than ours; if he is moved to a new home where the scent of other pets lingers, he may require time to connect and claim it as his new territory.

Animals may faintly sense the former pets' presence and possibly their desire to return. Cats especially have difficulty with change and need some time to reorient themselves and settle into their new environment. They will be initially exploratory, cautious, and even afraid. Pineapple helps them to "land" in their new environs.

Animals who have grown up in kennels or foster homes will also benefit from Pineapple Essence. In fact, this remedy is good for any pet raised in an environment that is temporary until he can be placed elsewhere.

Pineapple Essence will also support your pet's healthy sense of pride in his accomplishments. His need for praise may indicate a previously unsupportive home, although it can also stem from his desire to simply be acknowledged. We cannot praise our animals too highly or too often. They love it—and the same principle, in fact, applies to people. The dog who races from side to side on the porch when the owner returns and the cat who lays his spoils of the hunt at the doorstep are both expressing a desire for approval. Pineapple Essence provides this confirmation of their skills.

Sometimes an animal's orientation in his home or on his property can be undermined through poor care or training from a previous owner. Pineapple Essence can help this pet reestablish his confidence. Excellent for show animals, this remedy helps an animal do his best in competitions, shows, and county fairs.

For the pet who simply seems unsure of himself, Pineapple Essence is strengthening. Charlotte, a timid thirteen-year-old house cat, responded well to this remedy. Her owner explained, "I don't know what happened to her before I got her, but she's been a very frightened cat—afraid to go out, afraid when anybody came to visit me. Since I have been giving her the flower essence, she seems to have lost some of that fearfulness. The other day when my daughter came to visit, Charlotte didn't run out of the house as she normally does." Although Tomato Essence would be the obvious choice for fear, we used Pineapple Essence for Charlotte's shying away from people who entered within her territorial boundaries. If she had not responded to the Pineapple Essence, however, Tomato would have been the next essence in her program.

When other animals on the property seem to undermine a pet's natural sense of confidence, Pineapple Essence calmly helps him to regain his place in the hierarchy of the household. Gracie, one feline in a home of three cats, was repeatedly hesitant around the other cats, shrinking from their advances even when they were kindly ones. The evening after receiving Pineapple Essence, she resumed her place in the bedroom, even with the two other cats on the bed. When the more aggressive cat advanced on Gracie, she stood her ground, refusing to back away as before. And when the dominant cat responded with gestures of affection, Gracie behaved likewise.

Pineapple Essence for Pet Owners: Self-assuredness

The owner in need of Pineapple is basically an insecure person. He may have financial worries and be concerned about being able to support either himself or his pet. Food and basic supplies may be amply present, but there may be a shortage of pet toys and other accessories that make the pet's life more entertaining, which is especially important for indoor animals or dogs confined to the home and yard. This situation is due not so much to the owner's actual financial inability to supply equipment but rather to his constant fear of lack—that he will not be able to replenish his funds once they are depleted. Even individuals who have a minor or moderate lack of belief in themselves and their abilities will benefit from Pineapple Essence.

A person in the negative Pineapple state may have career problems or feel undervalued or underpaid at work. His self-doubt fosters a certain confusion about his ability to care for himself or others, including his pets. His inferiority complex will tend to magnetize the very shortage of resources that he fears. Other people get raises, he observes glumly, and have the homes and cars they want, but not him.

An insecure pet owner creates uneasy pets. Animals in the negative Pineapple state sense when their owner doesn't know where his next meal is coming from, and since they depend on him for their sustenance, his uncertainty affects their lives. Animals will become unsure of their own abilities; it may take longer to train them, or they may need to be retrained fairly often. Once the self-assured quality of Pineapple is returned to the owner's life, everyone can relax.

Raspberry Essence for Animals: Kindheartedness

Raspberry Essence supports a pet's natural tendency toward compassion. Animals can abandon themselves to love in ways to which people usually only aspire. Their sense of selflessness is the basis for many heroic stories of their compassion expressed, their forgiveness expounded. Horses in particular resonate with this remedy, as they have a profound ability to connect with their riders. For this reason, there are now a number of therapeutic riding centers for disturbed children.

The negative Raspberry state is characterized by a certain lack of sensitivity. Females of the Bengal cat breed, for example, are commonly known to be unforgiving and great grudge-holders. By nature strongly self-involved, cats relate everything back to themselves in an almost egoic way, for it is the ego that becomes offended when it feels slighted. Also rich in emotional fabric, these noble darlings can easily be put off or feel hurt. Grape, for feeling replaced by other cats or people, as well as Date, for getting irritated by the behavior of others in their space, all overlap in their application for felines. And since cats react so sensitively to harsh discipline, Raspberry Essence helps to heal their wounded spirits.

Animals who lash out through their behavior—be it barking, hissing, soiling, or shredding of furniture—may be asking for this essence. Pets whose play expresses a marked viciousness are, in their own way, in need of Raspberry's help. When their actions exhibit a tangible element of resentment, Raspberry Essence helps dissolve any lingering memory of mistreatment, no matter how subtle.

If not for outright meanness, Raspberry Essence is comforting to the animal who seems to have hurt feelings. This is a common remedy for domesticated animals who are so easily and often misunderstood, even by the most sensitive of owners. Although pets as a rule do not hold on to grudges, any physical or emotional hurt can affect their behavior. Some animals will feel hurt if not given enough attention; others will withdraw in quiet resentment if they see more energy being given to other pets in the household. Even pets who seem fine can enjoy the extra attention that giving them an essence, and especially Raspberry, provides.

Reilley, a mixed terrier breed, showed aggressive behavior in addition to barking on a virtually nonstop basis. According to his owner, he tended to bully the other dogs in his household, until he was given Raspberry Essence. Within four days, the barking had nearly stopped. "One morning," his owner commented, "I realized that Reilley barked but then stopped instead of barking continually. He's a tough nut to crack. This dog was hurt when I first got him. When I began putting the drops on his head, he lowered it all the way to the floor. This is a sign of respect. When you have a difficult dog, he will look you in the eyes a lot to challenge you. If he lowers his gaze, then he's submitting or showing respect. Reilley has always stared, always been aggressive until now."

Raspberry Essence for Pet Owners: Kindheartedness

Raspberry-deficient owners, out of their immense kindness and connection to their pets on a heart level, will sometimes feel responsible for their pet's pain or discomfort. "If only I had not let him out," they might say. Self-blame serves no one. A more constructive response would be to turn the Raspberry Essence's kindly forgiveness toward oneself.

For people who tend to be unforgiving of others, this essence is virtually imperative. Many individuals carry lifelong grudges toward their parents or other close family members that weigh them down as the years pass. Perhaps a parent was abusive, alcoholic, or otherwise neglectful. The personality defects in others are never excuses for holding grudges; they present all the more reason to forgive these parents who, themselves, were probably mistreated by their own kin. Once the people in need of Raspberry Essence learn the lesson of forgiveness, they will find others responding to them in vastly different ways—with kindness.

Owners with fiery tempers often express themselves harshly due to deeply unhealed emotional wounds. If not from parents and family, bitterness over difficult love relationships may often be the cause. Once we learn that the way we treat others matters more than how they treat us, we can begin to reclaim the state of mind we so desire—one that is loving, forgiving, and kindly.

It is important for pet owners needing Raspberry Essence to deal with these related issues; if unable to keep their emotions in check, they may vent their frustrations on their animals. Even a harsh word, to some species, can be devastating. And although this is not always the case for people in the negative Raspberry state, it is common enough to be worth mentioning.

For owners who are considering unnecessary euthanasia or any damaging and irreversible surgeries for their animals—such as declawing or debarking—in order to have their pets conform to domesticated life, Raspberry Essence is recommended. This remedy can help to open the heart's natural compassion and encourage them to seek less drastic solutions to treatable, trainable problems.

Spinach Essence for Animals: Simplicity

Spinach can assist your pet with the many stresses resulting from domesticated life. Animals who have started out in life as strays; pets who are highstrung and prone to stress; and animals who have been abused, abandoned, or neglected, especially in early life, respond beautifully to Spinach Essence.

Imagine yourself on vacation in a foreign country where the language, customs, food, and daily routine are completely unfamiliar to you. This parallels the dilemma faced by domesticated animals, whose natural habitat is the rugged outdoors. Domestic life versus existence in the wild are as night and day to each other. Therefore, the more you can create the most natural environment possible for your pet, supplemented by Spinach Essence, the happier and healthier he will be.

Spinach will also help your animal companions to relax in a stressful home. As previously mentioned, veterinarians concur that animals mirror, and also absorb, the emotional climate of their household. They pick up both the positive and negative emotions in their environment. Conversely, if alcohol or other abuses are present, we will see a troubled or anxious pet. And as they are so attuned to their owners' lives, the loss of a job, a child, or a marriage partner will be upsetting and anxiety-producing for pets in the household as well.

For the younger animal who acts older than his actual years—listless, disinterested in his surroundings, and sluggish in his digestive and eliminative habits—Spinach is an excellent aid. Please note that it is important to rule out any physical causes which may require medical attention; proper veterinary care is irreplaceable. And in addition to flower essences, all animals need a wholesome diet, exercise, rest, and love to improve the quality of their lives.

Spinach Essence is a wonderful supplement for older animals as well. For show or competition animals, including race horses, who are past their prime or have been "put out to pasture," Spinach helps to restore their sense of playfulness, adventure, and natural propensity for exploration.

For animals who have recovered from the trauma of surgery or serious illness but have not regained their interest in life, Spinach is recommended. One little poodle who had fully recovered from an accident and resultant surgery but "wasn't quite himself," according to his owner, had begun acting like a much older dog. "I gave him Spinach, and he started running and running around the table and playing with his little toys. He acted like a puppy again—playing, jumping, and seeing everything as a game." Acting old before their time is a completely correctable behavior in our pets. Our testimonials show that pets who mope and have lost their enthusiasm for life respond quickly—within mere days at most—to Spinach Essence.

Spinach Essence for Pet Owners: Simplicity

An individual lacking in the positive qualities of Spinach Essence has a strong propensity toward stress. The responsibilities of work, home, and family life will rest heavily on him, mainly due to a lack of trust that things will work out. He is the classic worrier.

Overly analytical and too much in his head, the individual needing Spinach Essence has lost the sense of rollicking fun so necessary to our physical and emotional well-being. Often, this individual has suffered through a dysfunctional childhood, colored by abuse, divorce, or alcoholism. He has had to work even harder at an early age simply to survive such an upbringing. These people have somehow lost the gift of childhood.

For this reason, they benefit enormously from sharing their lives with animals. In untold ways, pets help replenish those lost years of fun and games. A walk with the dog or even watching the goldfish for a short while will give perspective to this pet owner. It is precisely because people lacking in positive Spinach Essence qualities gain so much from caretaking pets that they can be so powerfully changed by their animals. The negative Spinach state, in other words, can be easily transformed by the right pet for this owner.

From the genus *Spinacea*, the tiny yellowish flowers of the bolted spinach plant emerge. Spinach is an annual of the goosefoot family, so classified for the shape of its leaves. Just as the hearty spinach plant requires a mere forty days to mature, so the negative Spinach state can be quickly dissolved in the company of fun-loving animals.

Strawberry Essence for Animals: Dignity

A lack of self-worth is a quality that does not apply to animals simply because they are not equipped with the faculty of self-consciousness. A pet will usually absorb this quality from a negative-state Strawberry owner or from being treated in ways that offend his innate and nature-given sense of dignity. Animals inherently know their worth; its absence is simply not an issue for them. Nature provides them with a healthy, adventurous sense of themselves; a keen interest in exploring; and an innate desire to aspire to a greater awareness of their inner joy.

Thus a pet's need for this essence can often be directly linked to the attitudes of the negative-state Strawberry owner who either treats his animals, or himself, with a marked lack of respect. And how can he do otherwise when he himself feels undeserving?

Pets who are difficult to train because they are grappling with basic issues of a healthy sense of themselves, projected onto them by their caregiver, can benefit from Strawberry Essence.

Strawberry is also the essence of choice for animals who are, literally, "on their last leg" and are nearing their own passing or in the midst of a lengthy period of recuperation. When independence-affirming actions are no longer within their capability—loss of bladder or bowel control, inability to walk, needing to be fed by others, or difficulty in grooming or otherwise caring for themselves—it is time for Strawberry Essence. The quality of dignity is paramount to animals as well as people.

In the following story, we see how a flower essence can reinforce an animal's innate sense of nobility. Although Tara, a twelve-year-old cocker spaniel, is relatively healthy, except for glaucoma and recurring bouts of bronchitis, she is a good candidate for Strawberry Essence. Called "the queen" by her loving owner, Tara "took to it immediately. She was attentive even before I opened the bottle. I know the dignity that it is giving her is excellent. I'm very thrilled with the results."

I remember many years ago seeing a goat who had just torn off half her udder on a barbed-wire fence. Her eyes had glazed over in severe shock, as a goat's udder is a vital anatomical center. Even so, it was with dignity that she continued grazing as though nothing had happened. Shock notwithstanding, instincts led her to a behavior that was both comforting and dignified. In this particular case, Pear would be the first essence in the goat's program, followed by Strawberry to help her ground herself once again.

Also, circumstances in the owner's life such as divorce or the leaving of a partner, or simply living in a household where the family is going through difficult times relating to one another, can warrant the pet's need for Strawberry Essence. These, too, are conditions that can destabilize an animal.

As Strawberry is the essence for grounding, it is helpful for pets who somehow feel that the ground has been taken out from under them. Cats, being especially territorial, are prime candidates for this essence. Any time they feel their space is threatened is an excellent time for this remedy, such as when other cats or animals are brought into the home or onto the property. Cleo, a large, bushy Persian cat, is a prime example. This feline was required to spend time in a household with a younger kitten, due to being boarded with a friend while her owner was absent on long business trips. Cleo expressed her sense of uprootedness by demanding attention from the owner, pushing the kitten out of bed, and bossing her away from the food bowls at mealtime. After two days on Strawberry, Cleo was sleeping in the same bed with the kitten, and the two were well on their way to becoming good friends.

Also, for pets who are simply needing to be more grounded in their bodies, Strawberry Essence is indicated. And whereas Avocado Essence will help animals achieve better mental presence, Strawberry offers an ability to be more solid in their personalities. Lucas, a three-year-old tabby tomcat, is a case in point. After one day on Strawberry Essence, he no longer ran from the sounds of rattling pans or people walking back and forth upstairs in his home. His owner described him as "more solid, stable, present, and confident."

Strawberry Essence for Pet Owners: Dignity

A Strawberry-deficient owner has difficulty seeing the nobility in anyone, including himself. The sad point here is that many people desperately need this essence, both in this country and globally. The reason so many people live unfulfilled lives is simply because they themselves feel they do not deserve to live otherwise. When I consult with clients, I find the need for this remedy surfacing repeatedly.

Strawberry-deficient owners often come from troubled homes themselves and have not been raised by role models who supported their sense of self-worth during their formative years. The beauty of this essence is its ability to mirror this lost dignity back to the owner. Pets can reflect back to an owner a glorious self-image of his own worthiness. For just as pets live in a sense of their place in this world, so do pet owners harbor an innate quality of expansiveness through the act of bringing pets into their lives.

Somewhat like Raspberry Essence for self-blame, Strawberry addresses the state of guilt. The difference between the two is subtle yet distinguishable. Blaming oneself is wasted regret; guilt is a sense of innate worthlessness. Both mental states have something in common—they are both a waste of time, are nonproductive, and prevent one from taking positive action when it is needed.

One pet owner shared that she blamed herself for the death of her cat. Seeing her cat across the street, she had opened the front door to let him in. While racing across the street, he was hit by a car. Finding him dead the next day in the neighbor's backyard, she spent two days torturing herself with guilt, feeling that she was responsible for his death—first, by opening the front door, and second, for not finding him soon enough to see that he received the care he required from the injury. She reported that Strawberry Essence was "like a balm for the heart."

Tomato Essence for Animals: Strength, courage

Tomato Essence is beneficial for any fear-based behaviors of either known or unknown origin. It is especially helpful for younger pets. The earlier in life they can learn attitudes of fearlessness—not to be confused with foolishness—the better.

One of my favorite "courage remedy" stories involves a longhaired gray tabby named Grasshopper who was given essences during her pregnancy. For a cat whose typical recreation consisted of chasing the deer out of the front yard where they regularly dined on fresh table scraps, her skittish behavior during pregnancy seemed clearly out of character. Any abrupt or piercing sounds made Grasshopper jump—the door inadvertently slamming, logs shifting in the fireplace, or loud voices echoing from the next room. Responding almost immediately to her "fear essence," Grasshopper completed the remainder of her pregnancy in a state of calm contentment. Some weeks later three of the most courageous kittens I have ever encountered were born. Usually the sound of a broom or vacuum is disturbing to newborns, but these kittens were extraordinarily fearless. To them, housecleaning implements were just another game. Oftentimes, too, little ones will dig their claws into the carpet when being lifted up. Not so with these kittens.

Visits to the vet are excellent opportunities to give Tomato to your cat, dog, or other pet. The sights, sounds, and smells of other unfamiliar animals, themselves afraid, can be frightening to your pet. If the visit is warranted by the need for emergency treatment, Pear is indicated as well, given alternately with Tomato rather than at the same time.

Many domesticated animals are traumatized by city life, a far cry from the feral existence of their ancestors. The sensory input to which we are so accustomed can easily evoke fear, or even terror, in our pets. These responses indicate the need for Tomato Essence. Some species, and particular animals within them, will handle transportation and relocation better than others. For cats in general, a move can be a severely traumatic experience. Unlike dogs, who are primarily people-oriented and thus coined "man's best friend," cats connect more to their environment. And for animals frightened in transport or refusing to enter a kennel, cage, or stall, Tomato proves calming and comforting.

Penny's story exemplifies the benefits of Tomato. Rescued by a kindly new owner from the animal shelter, this mixed breed of dog sported one bruised eye, several missing teeth, and patches of fur absent from her coat. Her behavioral symptoms included a fear of children and sounds such as doorbells and loud parties. Penny's first days in her new home were spent solely in eating and sleeping. Within days of being given Tomato Essence, she became more alert and assertive. Fear symptoms disappeared from her behavior. "Penny has since become a regular little guard dog," her owner reported, "barking when someone knocks at the door and patrolling the garden. She has also befriended the neighbor's dog. Before the Tomato Essence, noises would cause her to shake, panic, and act as if the world were about to end."

For animals bullied by other pets in the household or barnyard and who become withdrawn or fearful, Tomato proves strengthening (see Grape for tempering aggressive animals). Especially if food bowls are shared and the timid pet is not allowed his portion by the more aggressive animal, it is time for Tomato. This essence is also reinforcing for any animal born the runt of the litter. For the little pet who can't hold his own or stand up for himself with his siblings, Tomato can help him to be less fearful and to find his rightful and respected place in the pecking order or hierarchy of the home.

For the pet who is cowering, skittish, or easily spooked, the gentle action of Tomato Essence affords clear, and often remarkable, results. A four-year-old black Lab's story typifies this remedy's application. Sammy had been fearful of virtually everything and everyone since being retrieved from the pound as a young dog. When Sammy and I first met, her owner had already wanted for quite some time to give her away or take her back to the pound to be put down—whichever she found easier. "I don't have time for you" was the underlying message to Sammy, who was then boarded with the woman's relatives.

Barking was but one of Sammy's many behavioral problems, which her owner had previously treated with a shock collar. After a time, however, this approach proved ineffective. (Such methods, at best, merely skirt the underlying cause of an animal's troubled behavior, which is exactly where the power and beauty of flower essence treatment lies.) On repeated occasions, the neighbors' loud voices would trigger Sammy's even louder barking, with resultant complaints from other neighbors. A single dosage of Tomato essence, gently rubbed into her gums, quieted her within minutes. The problem, I am told, has not repeated itself.

Sometimes animals will attack out of fear and an instinctive sense of self-preservation. With horses in particular, their best defense is an offensive attack to protect their sensitive underbellies from possible predators. Tomato Essence will not eliminate an animal's common-sense need to defend itself, but it will help prevent any excessive or unnecessary fear. Fear of the outdoors or of new experiences in general is treatable with this remedy as well.

Tomato need not be administered for fear alone but also simply to strengthen your pet. For animals whose jobs include guarding and serving people, such as seeing-eye dogs and police dogs, this essence is useful.

Also, for animals who express anxiety during electrical storms and other extreme weather conditions and harsh seasons, this essence is indicated. Many are the fears that your pet may experience—some of them described in this section. Tomato is an important remedy to have on hand to fortify his inherent strength in the face of life's daily hardships, dangers, and difficulties.

Tomato Essence for Pet Owners: Strength, courage

Those in the negative Tomato state are fearful rather than worried, and weak rather than simply hesitant. A vast array of fears can attack us—of known and unknown causes—of events that have frightened us earlier in our lives, of experiences that have been painful in the past and present themselves again for us to face. Sometimes we may become overwhelmed by too many difficulties at once, or we are simply afraid to tackle the tests that lie before us.

Tomato-type challenges can be great or small in nature, frequently recurring or one-time-only tests. Either way, the lesson they present is to realize that we are inherently powerful and fearless and to bravely face any challenge, no matter how looming or difficult it appears. Fear of accidents, of flying in planes, of natural disasters such as earthquakes or floods all indicate a need for Tomato Essence.

Tomato also addresses issues of addiction to smoking, to overeating, and even to remaining in an unhealthy relationship. The pet owner in need of this remedy may have to develop his faculty of willpower to overcome his faults lest they impair the harmony of the household. If this essence is seriously needed for the owner, it will often be reflected in the troubled behavior of pets in the same home.

The Tomato-deficient pet owner needs to address his issues as best he can, with the support of this remedy. Otherwise he may easily pass his fears on to the animals in his household. Our pets are living conduits of our energy, thoughts, and emotions. The healthier we are, the happier they will be.

The tomato plant was once grown for its ornamental beauty alone. Throughout history, it acquired a reputation—biochemically unjustified— as an aphrodisiac and thus received the title of "love apple." In the non-lusty sense of loving, we could say that the tomato, in flower essence form, carries a message of the ability to love heroically.

In Conclusion

"Man is related to all nature," said Ralph Waldo Emerson. Mother Nature, in her kindness, has given us remedies for our ills. This world, it seems, is determined to set us off balance and out of sorts with Nature's strength and beauty. Through the study of plot-essence application for pets and animal enthusiasts, the importance of flower essences becomes increasingly apparent. It is here that we see the value of these remedies in restoring positive states once they are lost. The suffering of an animal that we love is surpassed in intensity by few things in our lives. We needn't worry; help is on the way through our love combined with the loving use of Nature's apothecary. With the tools of flower essences, we can set about making our animals more comfortable and, ideally, help them return to their natural state of balance.

Chapter Summary Outline

1. Essences needed by a person or pet who is not expressing the positive aspects of those remedies are called *plot* essences.

2. Plot essences are divided into two categories: *pivotal*, meaning with a life-long and frequently recurring need; and *peripheral*, used in specific situations, usually infrequent in occurrence.

3. Flower essences do not manipulate or control behavior.

4. An understanding of the animal's natural guidance by instinct assists in proper essence selection. Essences will not override their instincts but rather temper them to suit the animal's domesticated lifestyle.

5. Often, pets and their owners are in need of the same essence program.

6. Matching a pet's theme with the owner's plot essence, or the pet's plot essence with the owner's theme, is a very workable combination of personalities.

7. In this chapter, each of the Master's Essences is defined in terms of plot applications for pets and owners alike.

7
WHEN A PET DIES

He prayeth well who loveth well
Both man and bird and beast.
He prayeth best, who loveth best
All things both great and small;
For the dear God who loveth us,
He made and loveth all.
Samuel Taylor Coleridge

Pet owners are courageous people. They open their hearts, form timelessly deep bonds, and then must say farewell to their "dearest of the dear" when death calls. Sometimes, there is simply nothing we can do to save an animal's life. At that point, it is time to let go. As one sage said, "I'd rather be hurt a thousand times than lose the capacity to love."

In this chapter, I will offer suggestions for using each of the twenty Master's Essences to comfort grieving pet owners and, hopefully, to help them move forward in their lives. Flower essences can assist the individual facing the passing of a pet; the person whose animal has died in the recent past; or the individual who, though his animal companion died many years ago, still harbors unresolved issues.

The essence program for the animal who is passing on is much more simple. Typically it is Pear, for inner peacefulness, especially if the animal has been in an accident and has sustained trauma. This essence will also help him deal with the unsettling emotions of his human guardians, who are usually quite distraught themselves as they prepare for their pet's transition. Pear Essence will help an animal to regain his composure and reestablish his connection with Nature's natural rhythms. Strawberry Essence, too, can help an animal to reclaim his nature-given sense of dignity as his time of passing approaches. (See "Strawberry Essence for Animals" in chapter 6.)

Pear can also offer vibrational solace to the owners in preparing for the passing of a pet. One woman phoned our office to say how profoundly Pear Essence had helped her family immediately before and after their cat's death. The nine-year-old calico had fallen off the roof and irreparably broken her back, gone into seizures, and subsequently was put to sleep. Pear comforted everyone involved.

Remember, animals deal with discomfort much differently than we do. Pain, to them, is simply another event in their existence. (However, if their suffering is ongoing, Orange Essence assists them in dealing with lingering difficulties.) Plus, nearly all animal communicators report the same thing: Animals are ready for their own passing and are basically fine with it. It is the grievously upset owners whom our pets are concerned about, as they will love and serve us until their last breath. They pick up on our worry, our unwillingness to let them go, and our fear about how we will continue without them. For these reasons, their passing provides us with one of the greatest possible lessons: unconditional love. The highest service we can render them as their time of transition approaches is to love them freely and to free them from any attachments we might hold within our own hearts and minds.

Much of our pain around a pet's passing is our concern about ourselves—how will we get by without our special friend; who, or what, will fill the void once he leaves us; how can we face day after day without his endearing company?

The way individuals deal with the subject of death is, to some extent, culturally defined. In India, for example, a greater acceptance and even celebration of a loved one's passing is the cultural norm. An elaborate ceremony generally accompanies the event, with much honoring and respect for an incarnation well lived. A strong belief in the continuation of life through its changing forms sustains the loved ones left behind. This is not to say that the departed person is not missed, but their acceptance of death, and lack of resistance to it in the greater scheme of life, mitigates the sense of loss.

Age, illness, or a serious accident can indicate that the time is nearing for our pet to leave this world, possibly confirmed by the veterinarian through lab work indicating, for example, kidney failure or a diagnosis of great discomfort for the animal due to terminal illness or a serious accident. We may have to watch our pet's existence prolonged through torturous medical procedures or, when all else has failed, face the option of euthanasia. Accepting the reality of the situation, based on a diagnosis that you believe accurate, is one necessary step. Facing the situation with a flower essence program for yourself can be a significant means of support. What is the best way to determine an essence program for ourselves? A good rule of thumb is this: Whichever essences we feel our pet needs as the time of his passing approaches are most likely the essences that we ourselves may find beneficial.

One owner phoned my office from upstate New York regarding her ten-year-old Pekinese. Having raised Fred since the age of eight weeks, she seemed unwilling to agree with the prognosis of terminal cancer. He would surely heal, she assured me. The woman then requested the following essences for him: Orange, to help him deal with the depression of his condition and physical pain; Blackberry, to remove any negative feelings around his possible passing; Cherry, for his typically grumpy temperament; and Raspberry, to counter any residual hurt that Fred might be experiencing.

And what a perfect essence program it was—for her: Orange, to comfort her in her grieving and deep sense of loss; Blackberry, to help with the denial inherent in her conviction that he would survive, despite the veterinarian's diagnosis of an animal in a tremendous amount of discomfort and pain; Cherry, for getting through the ups and downs of recovering from the loss of a pet; and Raspberry, to forgive herself for feeling responsible for his illness, any regrets about her care for him, and the emotional hurt of his imminent absence from her life.

The experience of a pet's passing gives us the opportunity to love without condition—one of life's greatest lessons—as animals love us. In his book *Autobiography of a Yogi*, Paramhansa Yogananda relates an illustrative story on this subject. Many years ago at his boys' school in Ranchi, India, twenty-five acres of land provided grazing for pets and wildlife alike. One such animal befriended the young Yogananda—a small fawn who was wont to sleep in his room and greet him with a loving nudge each morning upon arising.

One morning, the master teacher left early for business in town. His unheeded warning to the students to not feed the deer, unfortunately, cost the animal's life. By the time he returned later that day, the nearly lifeless animal lay slumped in a heap. Beside himself with sorrow, Yogananda prayed fervently for the deer's life to be spared. In response, the animal stood on feeble legs and rallied his tiny form to respond.

Later that night in sleep, he dreamt of the deer, who prayed to be released from his pained body. Awakening at the moment of agreement with the dream-deer's plea, Yogananda found the little fawn dying. Thus he recognized the selfish nature of his attachment to the animal, expressed through his prayers that the deer remain with him, and was then able to release his hold on the little fawn's life.

We, too, can hold our animals back. Entire books have been dedicated to the subject of pet loss. And since we outlive our animal friends by many years, we may experience the death of many animals within our own lifetimes. Well-meant phrases like "Well, you had him for a long time" or "You can just get another one" offer little comfort.

Pets grieve deeply as well when their friends die, both animal and human. Tasha, a seven-year-old husky, suffered immensely when one of her owners passed away. Gone were the long walks in the countryside and the many hours they had shared in the garden. Listless and moping, head and tail cast downward, Tasha began virtually living at a neighbor's home that same week. After two days on Grape Essence, her owner reported, she had perked up and would lick the drops out of his palm.

Pets express their grief over lost animal friends with a variety of behavioral clues. One mother of three children recently phoned her veterinarian saying that she could no longer tolerate their two-year-old border collie's new behavior. Her concern for the safety of her family, visiting children, and strangers prompted her to admit that she was ready to give him away. Formerly a loving and watchful playmate for the entire family, the dog had become grumpy and unpredictable, even nipping at one of the children. The veterinarian then queried her about the dog. It happened that their old Doberman pinscher, who raised and befriended the collie, had passed away at the same time his behavior turned aggressive. This situation presented the perfect dynamic for flower essence application, particularly Grape Essence, though Orange Essence is also helpful for grieving. Pets need more loving care when their animal companions pass on, as this story illustrates.

Euthanasia

Euthanasia is a Greek word meaning "good, or merciful, death." Sometimes we are confronted with this option for our beloved animal companions. For many people, euthanasia is one of the hardest issues they will ever have to face. If these animals were not in our domesticated care, instinct would tell them when the time had come to walk off into the woods. Or, in their weakened and infirm condition, predators would be the natural cause of their demise. Through our intervention and advances in medical technology, pets today often face the possibility of life spans extended far beyond their natural years. Many people feel that, since we take responsibility for their lives, we must sometimes do likewise for their passing.

It may be time to allow an animal to move on if prolonging his life involves any or all of these procedures: repeated overnight hospital visits; injections or forced medications; multiple surgeries; or frequent trips to the veterinarian's office that, for some animals, are traumatic in themselves. Maintaining a sense of dignity is important to an animal, expressed through his ability to remain independent in feeding and evacuating. Being able to relocate from place to place without assistance—as locomotion is one of the primary distinguishing features of the animal kingdom—fosters an animal's innate sense of dignity.

Here are twelve suggestions to help pet owners face the possibility of euthanasia and to mentally and emotionally prepare themselves for the experience. Many of these issues also apply to the natural passing of a pet.

1. Has everything possible been done medically through a veterinarian whom you trust?
2. Have you gotten a second opinion if you felt it was necessary to do so?
3. Are you prepared to say good-bye to your pet?
4. If not, why? What can you do to prepare?
5. Is every household member included in the decision and able to prepare as well?
6. Is the animal's condition severe and irreversible and such that his life would be seriously compromised or incapacitated if he were to remain alive?

7. Would he still be able to walk, retain the faculty of his senses, and maintain control of evacuation?
8. Will the extension of his life, possibly by medical means that are sometimes costly and uncomfortable, be worth the suffering it will cause him? Or you?
9. Have you done everything you could for your pet to avoid the if-only-I'd-done-it-differently syndrome?
10. Do you have a special ceremony or service planned to commemorate his passing?
11. Do you have spiritual or religious beliefs to turn to for solace and inspiration?
12. Are there friends or support groups with whom you can connect?

One of my long-term clients and a rescuer of abandoned cats and dogs called one evening in tears. Her thirteen-year-old cat had reached the final stages of struggling with stomach cancer. The veterinarian could offer no other options; euthanasia seemed the only solution. She placed the cat on Pear Essence to comfort him, herself taking Grape Essence the night before and on the morning of his passing. "I never could have gone through this without the Grape," she explained. "He passed peacefully and is no longer suffering so terribly."

Flower Essence Assistance and Essence Enhancers

It is quite natural and understandable for a grieving pet owner to experience many emotions—such as anger, denial, and depression—as he comes to terms with the passing of a dear friend. And although guilt is not exactly an emotion, many people experience this self-blaming state. If not properly handled, these powerful feelings can be damaging to the owner as well as those at whom he directs them. For instance, the veterinarian or the driver of the vehicle that may have caused the accident to the animal are easy targets for vented anger. With some reflection and the aid of a flower essence program, the owner may be able to see that these people are themselves saddened by the loss of the animal. Anger may then be replaced by forgiveness; denial, by calm acceptance; depression, by joyful gratitude; and guilt, by a healthy clearing of self-negation.

People innately understand the power of ritual as an opportunity to collect their feelings, establish a sense of closure, and come to terms with significant events of joy and sorrow alike. Many people find comfort in a ceremony for their deceased pet. In honor of the depth of the pet/owner relationship, one can now find pet condolence cards in card shops. Along these lines, an official commemoration day entitled Pet Memorial Day—the second Sunday of every September—has been created by the International Association of Pet Cemeteries.

Another means of recovering from the grief of a pet's passing is the use of natural remedies. The following section listing essences for owners to take when their pet dies also illustrates the basic philosophy of flower essences: Treat the personality, not the symptoms. The symptom, in this case, is the pet's passing. Although we can always suggest Grape Essence for this issue, each individual—according to his particular temperament—will deal differently with the grieving process. Here, you will be able to see what essence, or essences, by definition match your special needs at this time. If several remedies seems appropriate, you may wish to prioritize them in order of immediacy for the single-essence dosage method. Or try a combination of several remedies if you are more comfortable with that approach.

In addition, I have suggested some supportive measures, entitled "Essence Enhancers," as a means of supplementing the remedies. These activities are designed to match the unique temperaments of each of the twenty Master's themes as well as the positive states of the essences themselves.

Almond: Self-control

Almond Essence helps the owner with excessive sadness to the point of obsession. When he cannot work through the grieving process but rather is consumed by it, Almond Essence is most helpful. Reliving the tragic parts of his pet's passing over and over is not. When his upset interferes with the rest of his life and his ability to function normally after a reasonable time has passed, this remedy helps to restore balance.

Essence Enhancers: Take a few deep breaths. Inhale calming memories of your pet; exhale disturbing thoughts. Allow yourself time for quiet activities of your choice that you find especially calming to the mind and nervous system.

Apple: Healthfulness

Apple Essence encourages the owner to resume a healthy lifestyle—to return to an exercise program, get lots of fresh air and sunshine, and basically get back to business as usual. Apple Essence reminds us that life goes on and that continued worry, fear, and doubt are injurious to health on all levels. This individual will be able to speak of his pet in conversation with healthy memories of their time together.

Essence Enhancers: Exercise! A good cardiovascular workout is known to help lift depression. Even if unwilling at first, many people report that once they get going, the benefits are practically miraculous and miraculously practical.

Avocado: Good memory

To remember a departed pet and to learn the lessons of our shared experiences with him is the message of Avocado Essence. That we are changed, that we have grown immeasurably through our interactions with each animal who has spent time with us, is a wonderful legacy to the richness of their friendships. Avocado helps us to integrate the precious experiences we have shared with our animal companion, enriching us as we move forward through each moment of every day.

Essence Enhancers: Put together a scrapbook of photos of your pet, or rearrange a book that you have previously compiled. If photos of your animal friend fill your home, you may want to put them in a special place to look at when you are prepared rather than seeing them when you may be caught off guard and have to struggle with still raw remembrances.

Banana: Humility

Banana Essence, with its calming quality of humility, gives us perspective on our pet's passing and on the re-creation of our lives as we move forward from that point in time. Banana Essence allows us to see the bigger picture and to understand the nature of suffering and death in a broader context. It depersonalizes the experience, thereby removing layers of our emotional pain. Some good questions to ask ourselves when taking this essence are, What suffers? What dies?

Essence Enhancers: If you have friends, family members, or co-workers who have recently lost an animal companion, send them cards of condolence and allow them the time to talk to you about their experiences.

Blackberry: Purity

Often, people can react negatively to the death of their pet. For people who interpret death in unfavorable terms, this essence can be of great assistance. Especially for those who say that they will never have pets again, Blackberry Essence helps remove the sense of pessimism or the focus on the difficulty of the situation. These thoughts are like shadows that pass with time and the use of Blackberry.

Essence Enhancers: The best possible support when taking this essence lies in repeating affirmations. You may either custom-design one for yourself in relation to your specific needs or repeat the following affirmation, first loudly with great will behind it, then more softly to draw it deeply into the mind, and finally mentally only with eyes closed: "Pure thoughts, harmonious actions. I see goodness everywhere and in all things."

Cherry: Cheerfulness

For the owner caught in bouts of moodiness after the passing of a pet, Cherry Essence is a helpful remedy. Notably if the moods seem to come and go, Cherry is indicated. The owner may feel temporarily OK in healing from his grief, and then another round of sorrow returns. Cherry provides a foundation of even-mindedness so that, eventually, the emotional heaviness will lift, replaced with a lighthearted cheeriness and pleasant memories of the departed pet.

Essence Enhancers: As Cherry Essence embodies the quality of cheerfulness, anything you can think to do that is light, fun, or playful will be a step in the right direction. Sing—even if you have to force yourself—in the shower, while doing laundry, while preparing meals. Dance—even if it feels unnatural—while running to the mailbox, the car, the bus stop. Lastly, if you can, whistle. It works.

Coconut: Upliftment

Coconut Essence is important for the pet owner shortly before the passing of his pet, especially if euthanasia is considered. This remedy helps the owner transmute his sense of imminent loss with the realization of the gift of his pet's companionship in the context of his own life. As the coconut grows many feet off the ground, its essence allows one an expanded, bird's eye view of the situation. Solutions are found in the very core of the problems they address; in this case, the owner finds an inner resolution within the context of his sorrow.

Essence Enhancers: The coconut tree grows in balmy climates, an image that leads the mind to thoughts of faraway, tropical vacations. Likewise, engage your mind in activities that disengage it, especially from its problem-oriented state. In other words, take a vacation from your regular mind-set. Go to the theater or cinema to watch plays or films with themes of heroism. Study the lives of people or animals who have championed against great odds.

Corn: Vitality

A perfect essence for helping the owner to face his future with energy and enthusiasm, Corn is the "moving forward" remedy. With respect for the natural grieving process and its timing, it is not so much that one needs to grieve for an expressed length of time but rather to deal with all the issues involved in the grieving process. The owner will find this essence helpful especially in cleaning out his departed pet's bedding and belongings, including toys, photos, and special mementos. With Corn Essence as a natural facilitator, the individual taking this essence may indeed find himself ready sooner rather than later to adopt a new friend. (Also see "Tomato Essence Enhancers.")

Essence Enhancers: Now is the time for new experiences, both outside and inside the home. Take up a new sport, take a day trip to a new place; or at home, remodel, rearrange, or splash on a new coat of paint.

Date: Sweetness, tenderness

Date Essence will help to replace the owner's sorrow with sweet remembrances of his beloved pet. As though piecing together a mental scrapbook

WHEN A PET DIES

of memories, Date Essence allows for a sense of closure. This remedy will also help the owner to relate to other animals as though they were members of his closest family. He can learn the lesson that having loved once, he can love deeply once again.

Essence Enhancers: Read stories of animals, even children's books, of breeds and species different from the departed pet. This will serve as a means of expanding your kinship with other animals. If it is not too painful, you can also practice an exercise of spotting a particular feature or quality in other animals whom you know that express some aspect of your departed friend. For the grieving pet owner who needs Date Essence, this is a time to reach out to others and to spend more time with family and friends and even neighbors with whom you have not yet become acquainted.

Fig: *Flexibility*

When a pet with whom we have intricately shared the ins and outs and the ups and downs of our daily existence is no longer around, many simple adjustments need to be made. The care we lavished is no longer required. For some people, adjusting their schedules causes renewed sadness or difficulty. Fig Essence supports the owner in making changes in his routine.

Essence Enhancers: Set up a new routine in your life to replace the one you previously shared with your pet. If feeding time was a special event, add something new in that time slot—a radio show, an inspiring lecture or book-on-tape, or a classical music program. Fill in that space in your daily planner with positive activities to which you can look forward.

Grape: *Love, devotion*

Grape Essence, as mentioned at the beginning of this chapter (see also "Grape" in chapter 6) is the classic essence for bereavement. Countless testimonials report the same experience: This essence helps people to understand the true nature of love, and it diffuses a personalized sense of loss. Much like Date Essence, it also helps us to see the endearing qualities of our deceased pet in other animals—a sparkle in the eyes of a newborn fawn or a certain way that the neighbor's dog wags his tale in expectancy of his owner's return.

Regardless of their individual temperaments, people in general experience grief over a pet's passing, resulting in the need for Grape Essence. Grape affirms that no love is ever lost. We can, in fact, continue loving our departed friend and express that gift of love over the years to come.

Grape Essence assists pets and people alike in recovering from bereavement, helping them to rebuild their lives in the absence of a lost loved one. Remember that when using Grape for these issues, one may need to remain on it over a period of time and possibly in several cycles as the grief returns.

Essence Enhancers: Whenever thoughts of the departed animal return to your mind, send out love to him. It may feel silly to say aloud, "I love you, Buddy," but grieving pet owners are allowed to do silly things. This is our opportunity to love more, not less, to remain open and not close down.

Lettuce: *Calmness*

On Lettuce Essence, excited emotions around the issue of a pet's passing can be put to rest and replaced with calm feeling. Lettuce represents the calm after the storm, the storm symbolizing the pain of loss. Lettuce will not suppress the natural grieving process. Quite the opposite—it merely smooths out the rough edges, allowing for a quiet reconciliation of the owner's deeper connection with his animal companion now gone.

Essence Enhancers: Any activity that calms the mind is recommended, such as yoga postures or tai chi movements. Meditation, too, is highly recommended. You may also want to create a sense of closure on the grieving process by writing an inspiring story about your pet, either for yourself or to share with others.

Orange: *Joy*

This is the classic essence for grieving and depression. A supportive measure while taking Orange Essence is to house-sit for friends and relatives with pets. This opportunity will allow you to keep your heart open to other animals; they can assist you through your healing process and communicate through their own joy that life, indeed, goes on.

Essence Enhancers: Do not allow yourself to dwell on any negative subjects related to your pet or his passing. Find little joys—watch other animals in the park or visit pet stores. Treat yourself to little things that amuse or entertain you; in temporarily releasing your mind from sadness, you can begin to build on the happiness you experience until it outweighs the times of sorrow.

Peach: Selflessness

Peach Essence, for mothering, is important in healing from grief over the loss of a pet. This remedy helps us to focus on others and their needs, which then frees the sadness from our minds and hearts. It is easy to lose perspective when a pet, with whom we may experience tremendous depths of undying love, is no longer around. Peach Essence helps to restore a sense of the expanse of the heart; like a bottomless well, it nurtures all who drink from it.

Essence Enhancers: Volunteer for special projects in your community or religious organization, if you feel drawn to do so. You may want to help out at the local animal shelter. If this is not an option, joining the Humane Society or an animal-rights group is another possibility. For more information, the Internet offers endless potential.

Pear: Peacefulness

Pear Essence is a classic emergency remedy to help the grieving owner reach a state of inner peace and calm resolution. Pear offers a vibrational message much like being patted on the back and told that everything will be OK. It helps to balance and harmonize any emotions that are still unsettled. "Rest in peace" is a saying not only for the departed animal companion but for those left behind.

Essence Enhancers: Long walks in nature, if possible, are a perfect supplement to Pear Essence. Just as animals are nurtured and restored through fresh air and brisk walks, so people can benefit from reconnecting with nature's healing essence.

Pineapple: Self-assuredness

Loss of a pet can be somewhat confidence-shattering, especially if the pet and owner were very close. This individual, to some extent, has defined his personality in relation to his pet. For the owner who feels that a part of himself has passed away along with his pet, Pineapple Essence helps one to "pick up the pieces" of his life. If or when he does want to adopt another pet, Pineapple can assist him in confidently selecting the right companion to match his lifestyle and household.

Essence Enhancers: If you are planning on bringing another pet into the household, this is the time to prepare for it—a larger pen, repair work on the fence, a new birdcage. Add as much creativity and personal style as you like.

Raspberry: Kindheartedness

Raspberry Essence helps the owner who blames himself after his pet's passing for improper caretaking while the animal was alive. This owner may somehow even feel responsible for his pet's death, either consciously or unconsciously. He may be heard to say, "If only I had done this or that." Raspberry helps the owner to forgive himself, gently accepting whatever has happened in relationship to his pet's last days.

Essence Enhancers: Get to know some of the neighborhood animals. Perhaps you can help with care and feedings while the owners are gone on vacation. The more you connect with them through eye contact—gently, not invasively—the more you will find a response in your own heart as it heals.

Spinach: Simplicity

Spinach Essence supports the restoration of a sense of playfulness and fun—both being signs of healing from the grieving process—and a childlike sense of the possibility of new adventures. This essence also addresses the owner's ability to trust that his pet had a wonderful sojourn with him, that his animal friend entered and exited his life at exactly the right moments.

Essence Enhancers: This is a perfect time for a trip to the zoo. To spend time in the company of other animals—especially to see the endless variety of bodies and behaviors—is a delightful treat. Also helpful is watching children at the zoo as they observe the animals.

Strawberry: Dignity

Strawberry Essence, with its ennobling qualities, helps the owner to regain his sense of poise and grace. When we lose a pet, we may often feel as though the ground were taken out from under us. Even as the luscious strawberry fruit grows low to the ground, this essence helps return our sense of grounding. Sometimes prolonged sorrow can obscure our own awareness of the beauty around us. Strawberry Essence allows us to see through these veils of sadness.

Essence Enhancers: Read books about heroic animals who have saved the lives of other animals, their owners, or even strangers. Focus on the nobility of spirit that leads them to such actions.

Tomato: Strength, courage

For the strength to endure great loss and to know that we will love animals again, and love them heroically, Tomato Essence is suggested. To face challenges and fears without their animal friends, these owners can learn the lesson of putting their lives in order. Especially for people who lose a treasured pet and then say that they will never again have animals in their household or on their property, Tomato Essence allows them to take the first tiny steps toward being open to adopting other pets.

Essence Enhancers: It may be time to consider another pet—possibly another species or a different breed. Remembering that we can never replace a departed friend, we can still take comfort in expanding our sympathies through loving again.

In Conclusion

We love, we lose, and the grief is real. In the case of deep loss, we tend to heal in stages. It is important to understand that flower essences do not take away the pain of our loss; they do, however, help us to live with and understand it better. Time, as the saying goes, heals all wounds.

Dogs and cats, studies have shown, require one to six months to adapt to a friend's passing, and it may take a year or more for people to heal from the death of a pet. If you are considering adopting another pet after the death of an animal companion, be sure to take Grape, or other essences in the list above, until the grieving has either lessened or subsided. Yes, the animals we lose are irreplaceable; they cannot be substituted by other pets. But we can love again. We can bring new pets into our home to care for. Pet stores, breeding establishments, rescue centers, shelters, and pounds abound with animals just waiting to love and be loved.

8

THE ANIMALS' GIFT TO US

The quizzical expression of the monkey at the zoo comes from his wondering whether he is his brother's keeper, or his keeper's brother.
Evan Esar

Clinical Evidence and Individual Case Reports

You have just read a book on improving the care of your animals. Their regard for us, as our own experience confirms, is exemplary; their healing effect on our behavior is practically miraculous. One of the more unusual studies conducted took place in Czechoslovakia to determine the effect of animal companions on individuals in long-term isolation. The data concluded that the company of animals is so vital to the physical and emotional health of humans that they should accompany people on space flights.

Recent studies show that pet owners are less likely than non-owners to contract heart disease. Plus, owners who have suffered heart attacks live longer than their non-pet-owning counterparts. In fact, animals in the home have been proven to be more effective for calming their hypertense owners than a leading blood-pressure medication. According to research at New York State University, married couples with pets report closer and more satisfying relationships as well as lower blood pressure under stress and following arguments than non-pet-owning couples.

Perhaps most impressive of all are the documented instances in which animals' natural heightened instincts allow them to predict seizures in their owners before they actually happen, alerting the people beforehand in sometimes life-saving situations. Cats, dogs, and even iguanas are some of the unlikely heroes in these stories. Pilot studies, with remarkably accurate results of nearly 100 percent, show that some dogs, due to their extrasensory olfactory abilities, are able to smell certain types of cancer—melanoma and lung cancer—at very early stages. In fact, the bloodhound—who tracks by scent alone and can follow a human trail for over fifty miles—is the only canine breed whose "testimony" is allowed in the United States judicial courts.

Several years ago, the American Veterinary Medical Association stated that sufficient clinical evidence and individual case reports exist confirming the benefits of alternative healing methods such as herbs, acupuncture, chiropractic, and homeopathy. Acupuncture, in fact, was recognized as "an integral part of veterinary medicine." One study in Venezuela reported that dogs who were given acupuncture along with antibiotics for ear infections recuperated significantly more quickly than those given only the medications. Recovery time was hastened; pain symptoms decreased notably.

One veterinarian, an adamant nonbeliever in the connection between emotional states and physical illness, recently received confirmation of this connection from an unlikely source—his own cat. An abandoned feline—covered with a persistent and unsightly skin rash—was dumped at his office by people who rightly presumed on his compassion. Since the cat's future looked bleak and homeless, he took it in. Much to his amazement, after several months in a stable home with no treatment other than regular doses of love, the cat's skin problem disappeared altogether.

A significant number of people have witnessed improvement in the quality of their pets' lives through alternative methods of treatment that recognize and address the body-mind relationship—combined, of course, with love. Two-thirds of Americans currently use holistic therapies for themselves and their families—why not for their pets as well? Since medical diagnosis of a pet's problem is clearly an integral part of pet care, a truly holistic approach need not be a question of one versus the other. In fact, holistic therapies complement standard allopathic treatment. Flower essences, more and more, are making their way into holistic care—for people and animals alike.

The following example from Rena Ferreira, D.V.M., illustrates this point: "An eleven-year-old springer spaniel was in for surgery to remove a large mass next to his rectum. These surgeries can be difficult no matter the age, but for this old fellow I was particularly concerned about his recovery. We used acupuncture needles to enhance anesthesia, allowing us to use less medication and inhalant, and also for post-op analgesia. As he was waking we could see he was very uncomfortable. Pear Essence was rubbed onto his ears and he settled right down into a nap. We kept the analgesic injection close by in case we needed to use it, but it did not become necessary."

Tools for Improved Pet Care

Children and animals as well as adult humans can appreciate the beauty of nature. Out for a walk, Calvin, of cartoon fame, discusses the fate of a dead bird in the path with Hobbes, his stuffed-tiger friend.

Contemplating the beautiful but expired life form before them, Calvin ruminates on the miraculous nature of existence—its fragility, temporal nature, and preciousness.

"It's very confusing," Calvin concludes. "I suppose it will all make sense when we grow up."

All too often when we do grow up, we become preoccupied with the demands and resultant stresses of existing in this world. Animals can link us back to nature. In so doing, they help us reconnect with ourselves.

The gifts that animals offer to this world are indeed far-reaching. In fact, one could even say they are faultless barometers of our behavior. Our relationship with animals, in this sense, gives us the opportunity to claim our highest potential as human beings. "The greatness of a nation and its moral progress," cited Mahatma Gandhi, "can be judged by the way its animals are treated."

Great people recognize greatness in the animal kingdom. In honor of its citizens, Albert Schweitzer has left us this humble legacy: "Hear our humble prayer, O God, for our friends, the animals. Especially for animals who are suffering; for any that are hunted or lost or deserted or frightened or hungry; for all that must be put to death. We entreat for them all Thy mercy and pity, and for those who deal with them, we ask a heart of compassion and gentle hands and kindly words. Make us, ourselves, to be true friends to animals and so to share the blessings of the merciful."

Anyone who has ever cared for pets—whether they be scaled, furred, feathered, or fleeced—knows from direct experience the joy and fulfillment they usher into our lives. Our animal friends, from mongrels to prize-winning purebreds, touch our hearts. We laugh at their mannerisms; we cry at their passing. Their accomplishments make us proud; their illnesses cause us pain. Our animal companions wait for us by the window, the gate, the barn door. They are there for us through thick and thin, through our rockiest ups and downs. Without attending a single self-help workshop, animals possess extraordinary relationship skills—they love without condition.

Flower essences allow us the opportunity to be there for them. These natural remedies help our animal friends to heal from accidents, illnesses, and surgeries. They restore our pets to healthy behaviors, dispelling their fears and needs. They assist gently, non-invasively and powerfully, without side effects. Flower essences are a significant, time-proven addition to the care we offer our animals.

Those who share with me their flower essence stories about their pets do so with animation, excitement, and enthusiasm. It is never "just a cat" or "only a dog" whose story they are recounting. It is a beloved, respected life companion. *Flower Essences for Animals* is not a book to convince you that animals deserve better care. Its purpose is to give you, a loving pet owner, the very tools with which to do it. Their enrichment of our lives is immeasurable; may we honor them a thousandfold in return.

Appendix

THEME QUALITIES AND BEHAVIORS

You will find listed in the following charts the identifying characteristics of each theme essence for both animals and pet owners. Some essences will overlap in a quality or two; Coconut and Avocado, for example, both catalogue the quality of alertness, and yet the overall picture for each of the two essences is quite different.

Theme Qualities and Behaviors of Animals

Almond
Calmness
Control in habits
Quietude
Balance
Moderation in all habits
Unobtrusiveness
Inwardly expressed personality
Contentment
Undemanding nature

Apple
Healthfulness
Exploration
Alertness
Glow of health
Joy of being in this world
Good-natured
Non-fretting
Healthy infancy
Functional childhood
Exercise-wise

Avocado
Good memory
Alertness
Lives in the moment
Inquisitiveness
Curiosity
Exploration
Responsiveness to training
Responsiveness to owner
Sophistication
Maturity
Awareness

Banana
Humility
Calmness
Easy companionship
Accommodating
Gentleness
Unassertiveness
Nondefensiveness
Good with children
Patience
A group participant

Blackberry
Purity
Innocence
Lack of guile
Sleek in appearance
Awareness of environment and others
Trusting companion
"The therapist"
Maturity

Cleanliness
Easily trained
Grooming-conscious
Offended by untidiness

Cherry
Cheerfulness
Entertaining personality
Even temperament
Easygoing nature
Youthfulness
Playfulness
Richness
Lightness
A sincere friend
Non-moodiness
Good-natured
Happiness

Coconut
Upliftment
Bright nature
Alertness
Transcendence
Adaptable nature
Gets along with others
Stamina
Perseverance

Corn
Vitality
Energy
Enthusiasm
Joy

Likes new experiences
"The adventurer"
Interest in new escapades
Happiness
Delight in abilities and environment

Date
Sweetness
Tenderness
Love
Embracing nature
Beauty
Nonjudgmental
Non-critical
Non-comparing
Specialness
Draws companionship

Fig
Flexibility
Acceptance
Relaxation
Easygoing attitude
Sense of comfort
Flowing personality
Adaptability

Grape
Love
Devotion
Healthy infancy
Adjusts well
Loyalty
Lifelong friend

Constancy
Commitment
Non-threatened nature
Fullness of personality
Dearness

Lettuce
Calmness
Strongly felt presence
Comfort-giving
Energy
Quietness
Undemanding
Non-needy nature
Good communicator
Contemplative nature
Reflective personality

Orange
Joy
Enjoyment
Companionship
"Sadness absorber"
Happiness
Untouched by grief
Resilience

Peach
Selflessness
Concern for others' welfare
Caretaker
Mothering nature
"Born nurturer"
Sharing nature

Good with children
Love
Trust

Pear
Peacefulness
"Emergency Essence animal"
"The healer"
Steadiness
Balance
Unflappable nature
Good in crisis
Comfort
Equanimity
Endurance of illness or injury
Connection to nature
Barometer of impending events
Calming effect on others
Positively changes people

Pineapple
Self-assuredness
Center of attention
Genuine, innocent pride
Cat bringing home prey
Dog guarding property
Charm
"Show-stopper"
Attractiveness
Attention-getting actions
Sense of own identity
Appreciation of praise
Intelligence
Expression of preferences

Raspberry
Kindheartedness
Friendliness
Comfort
Sensitivity
A feeling nature
Good with people, especially children
"Reads energy"
Deep bonding
Eye contact
Expressive eyes
Responsive eyes
"A good listener"
Nonjudgmental
Non-resentful

Spinach
Simplicity
Delight
Innocence
Trust
Playfulness
Fun-loving spirit
Relaxation
Stress-free character
Soothing personality
Helps with "lightening up"

Strawberry
Dignity
Grace
Nobility
Poise
Sophistication

Quietude
Sense of own beauty
Maturity
Royalty
Expression of preferences
Refinement of character
Charm
Embarrassment with training errors
Worth-affirming

Tomato
Strength
Courage
Instinctual intelligence
Guard dog
Natural rescue animal
Seeing-eye dog
Police dog
Upright posture
Welcoming of life
Facing difficulties
"Sixth-sense animals"
Saving lives
Alerting people to danger

Theme Qualities and Behaviors of Pet Owners

Almond
Self-control
Calmness
Inconspicuousness
A homebody
Availability for pets
Easygoing nature

Comfortable companion
Moderation
Balance

Apple
Healthfulness
"Health nut"
Nutritionally informed
Stamina
Sports participant
Sensitivity to pet's need for health

Avocado
Good memory
Avid interest in learning
Knowledgeable as a pet owner
Joy in gathering knowledge
Focused mind
Alertness
Concentration
Reader of pet's body language and other clues
Astuteness
Inventiveness
A natural explorer

Banana
Humility
Calmness
Kindness
Gentleness
Non-identification with own ego
Creates an unemotional household
Relaxation
Lack of self-absorption

Impersonal nature
Unimposing personality
Shares home easily with pets

Blackberry
Purity
Principled
Well-educated
Insightfulness
"The counselor"
A good friend to talk to
Cleanliness
Kindly sense of humor
Dislike of negativity
Straightforwardness
Non-ambivalent training of pets

Cherry
Cheerfulness
Childlikeness
Lightheartedness
Bubbliness
Laughter
Smiles
Joking nature
Fun-oriented
Even-mindedness
Good-natured personality
Stability
Match for rambunctious animals
Good with younger pets
Playfulness
Impersonal nature

Coconut
Upliftment
Improvement-oriented
Problem-solving orientation
Works through obstacles
Awareness
"Quality time" with pets
Bonds with animals
Learns from pets

Corn
Vitality
Energy
Not blocked by negative patterns
Non-procrastination
Good pet care
Exercise
Improvements on facilities
Consistency of energy

Date
Sweetness
Tenderness
Acceptance
A "safe" friend
Not easily irritated
Makes friends readily
Embracing nature
Buying presents for pets

Fig
Flexibility
Self-acceptance

Fluidity
Adaptability
Good traveler and companion
Openness
Comfort in different environments
Easygoing nature
Blends energy with pets

Grape
Love
Devotion
Connection with animals
Relates deeply to others
Intuition
Nurturance
Acceptance
Befriending others
Patience
Good with previously abused animals

Lettuce
Calmness
Quietness
Retiring nature
Highly creative
Good communication skills
Innovative personality
Calming to the emotionally agitated
A comfort to pets
Not upset over animal problems

Orange
Joy
Characteristic smile

Sustains through difficulties
Adored by pets
Fullness in energy
Raising happy pets
Gladness

Peach
Selflessness
Concern for others
Communication
Understanding of pets
Senses needs of animals
Nurturance
Serviceful quality
Serves needs of pets

Pear
Peacefulness
"Emergency Essence" personality
Mellowness
Comfort
Values animals
Solidity
Firmly rooted personality
Integration of people with pets
Owner of more than one breed or species

Pineapple
Self-assuredness
"Life of the party"
Eccentricism
Individualism
Definite ideas on many issues
Charisma

Exuberantly refreshing
Respects pet's individuality

Raspberry
Kindheartedness
Embracing quality
Compassion
Sensitivity
Sympathy
Empathy
Good listener
Understanding
Ideal pet owner
Concerned and caring owner
Good owner for previously mistreated pets

Spinach
Simplicity
Childlikeness
Fun
Playfulness
Enjoyment of children's activities
Straightforwardness
Trustworthiness
Honesty
Healthy childhood
Excellent pet owner

Strawberry
Dignity
Grounding
Responsible nature
Refinement
Owner of purebreds

Praise-lavishing with pets
Earthiness
Elegance
Graciousness
Generosity
Poise
Empowering companion
Pampering by nature

Tomato
Strength
Courage
"Brave warrior"
Energy
Stamina
Willpower
Faces obstacles
Forthrightness
Willingness to be wrong
Loving but firm disciplinarian
Breeder of fearless animals
Gallantry
Ability to adopt another pet when one has passed on

PLOT QUALITIES AND BEHAVIORS

The following charts list the plot qualities—those traits, problems, and weaknesses which indicate that an essence is needed by animals and pet owners. Both pivotal and peripheral plot indications are listed here. There is often an overlap in the plot qualities for pets and their owners as shown in these charts. (For a more complete explanation of plot essences, please see chapter 6.)

Plot Qualities and Behaviors of Animals

Almond
Lack of calmness
Being out of control
Lack of adjustment to domesticated life
Need to learn balanced living
Need for moderation
Overweight
Stress
Remaining indoors when accustomed to roaming free
Nervousness
Caginess
Nervous marching, or pacing
Out of sync with natural rhythms
Overgrooming
Chewing
Gnawing self or objects
Obsessive destruction of property
Frenetic habits
Obsessive behaviors

Apple
Consciousness of health
Imminent illness
Recovery from illness

Sense of weakness and vulnerability
The runt of the litter
Need for robustness
Need for adjustment to infirmities
Bad or unhealthy behavior
Health-related fears passed on through the owner
Owner-induced worry
Owner-caused doubt
Reinforcement of owner's fears

Avocado
Poor memory
Dreaminess
Unresponsiveness
Unfocused energy
Failure to come when called
"The roamer"
Loss of interest in life
Loss of a companion
Loss of life direction
Need for support in training
Need for sharper learning skills
Need for alertness
Need for the ability to retain information
Lack of focus
Slow learner
Speeding learning skills for intelligent animals

Banana
Lack of calmness
Overly emotional behavior
Excessive displays of negative behavior
Moodiness
Excessive agitation

Becoming inappropriately riled
Gentleness and sensitivity
Reinforcement of positive behaviors
Non-aggressiveness

Blackberry
Sense of uncleanliness
Absorption of the owner's negativity
Unhealthy human role model
Negative temperament
Inability to groom oneself
Inability to care properly for oneself
Need for ability to deal with difficult physical conditions
Need for cleanliness in soiled or sprayed-on areas
Exposure to harmful chemicals

Cherry
Cheerlessness
Moodiness
Contrary behavior
Orneriness
Grumpiness
Bad-tempered nature
Being a "sourpuss"
Need for loving guidelines and parameters
Need for honoring of pet's preferences
Need for setting comfortable boundaries
Spoiled
Mirroring the owner's needs
Troubled feelings

Coconut
Stuck in difficulties
Need for support of animal's desire to evolve

Chronic pain issues
Need for finding comfort in physical discomfort
"Creakiness" in the limbs
"I can't" attitude
Need to "stand up for themselves"
Transcendence of weaknesses
Sense of limitation
Loss of a companion

Corn
Lack of energy
Need for restoration of a sense of adventure
Relocation to a new home
Need for adjustment after a move
Withdrawn behavior after a move
Need for integration
Need to explore
Need to investigate
Lack of enjoyment
Upset from rearranging furniture
Difficulty with change
Need for renewed interest in life
Need to spark curiosity
Lack of zest for new experiences
Being a "couch potato"
Sluggishness in the owner
Old age
Loss of "spunkiness"
Need to be perkier and peppier
Exhaustion

Date
Sour disposition
Orneriness

Feistiness
Having an "off" day
Crabbiness
A picky nature
Irritability
Expressions of dislikes and disfavor
Picking on other animals
Lack of sweetness

Fig
Rigid nature
Incorrect training
Feeling somehow "not OK"
Feeling his behavior is unacceptable to the owner
Owner-related problems
Lack of consistent, firm, loving discipline
Mixed messages from owner
Confusion
An unknown past history
Confusion by too many rules
Uncertain of own behavior
Unsure of acceptable behavior
Lack of adaptation to too many rules
Fussiness
Intolerance of food
Whininess
Discontentment
Need for adjustment
Need for training
Need for breaking existing bad habits
Variations in eating or sleeping habits
Alterations in established routines
Changes in the home
Changes in ownership

Grape
Lack of love
Needy behavior
Abandonment
Jealousy toward other people in household
Jealousy of other household animals
Showing expressions of disapproval
Whining or crying for no apparent reason
Being forgotten
Loss of interest in food
Severing of ties with people or animals
Loneliness
Clinging behavior
Aloof or withdrawn nature
Bullying behavior
Overly or inappropriately territorial behavior
Mean-tempered or dangerous behavior
Listlessness
Unapproachableness
Bereavement, grieving
Loss of an owner or animal friend
Neglect
Soiling
Spraying or marking

Lettuce
Restlessness
Youthful immaturity
Short attention span
Lack of focus
Need for removal of distractions
Tension
Agitation
"Going nuts"

Wound-up behavior
Need for accommodation of new energies
Emotionally-based lack of calmness
Anger

Orange
Unhappiness
Depression
Abandonment
Abuse
Neglect
Loss of companion
Loss through death
Loss through relocation
Need for adaptation to indoor life
Listlessness
Despair
Weakened immune system
Magnified propensity toward illness
History of multiple homes
Depressed owner
Ongoing illness
Injury
Declawing
Debarking
Unnatural altering for domestication
Hormonally-based depression
Needing help during pregnancy or after birth
Long birthing sessions
Grieving
Setbacks
Relapse of illness
Battle with terminal illness
Ongoing physical infirmities

Exhaustion
Being pushed past limits
Loss of spirit
Emotional struggle

Peach
Self-involved
Overly demonstrative
Following owner around
Premature weaning
Drooling
Clawing as though nursing
Grown animals trying to nurse on other animals
Chewing or suckling on furniture or clothing
Emotional dependence
Demanding
Not "getting it"
Over-possessive
Insistence on meals before feeding time
Excessive territorialism
Having one's babies given away
Temporary separation
Visits to the veterinarian
Loss of young
Feeling threatened by younger pets in the household
Need to relax territorial instincts
Need to get along with other pets in the household
Embracing quality
Expansive nature

Pear
"Emergency Essence"
Need to restore peace and equilibrium
Boarding

Nervous and needing to be calmed
Birthing
Transportation
Disturbance of normal routine
Changes in feeding schedule
Insecurity
Instability
Panic
Anxiety
Disorientation
Pacing and calling (horses)
Accidents, injuries, or surgeries
Injured and left overnight at the hospital
Upsets due to illness
Support with allopathic or other medications
Crises
Shock or trauma
Biting
Scrapes, bruises, or falls
Wounds (surface or puncture)
Bites and stings (ticks, spiders, snakes, and insects)
Burns and heat stroke
Approaching death

Pineapple
Insecurity
Weak sense of identity
Living in households with children or other animals
Living with lingering scent of previous animal occupants
Difficulty with change
Cautious behavior
Fearful behavior
Raised in a kennel or foster home
Living in temporary housing

Unsupportive home environment
Undermined orientation to home or property
Poor care or training
Show animals needing to present their best images
Unsure of self
Shying away from people
Lack of confidence
The runt of the litter

Raspberry

Mean-spirited nature
Insensitivity
Unforgiving nature
Grudge-holding nature
Reaction to harsh discipline
Lashing out
Barking
Hissing
Shredding of furniture
Viciousness expressed in play
Resentment
Memory of mistreatment
Hurt feelings
Misunderstood
Withdrawn
Resentful of affection shown to other pets
Aggression
Soiling
Spraying or marking

Spinach

Stress of domesticated life
Having been a stray
High-strung nature

Abuse
Neglect in early life
Surviving in a dysfunctional and stressful household
Absorbing emotions of household
Alcohol in the home
Listlessness
Sluggish bodily habits
Loss of interest in environment
Acting older than one's years (when young)
Acting old (when old)
Being "put out to pasture"
Brooding nature
Lack of fun and playfulness
Recovery from trauma of surgery

Strawberry
Lack of worth
Living with a negative-state Strawberry owner
Having one's dignity offended
Owner-related problems
Difficulty in training
Non-healthy sense of self projected by caregiver
Approaching death
Lengthy recuperation time
Loss of bladder or bowel control
Inability to walk
Needing to be fed by others
Difficulty in grooming or caring for oneself
Needing grounding
Divorce or separation of partners
Difficulty in the household
Instability
Threatened territory
Uprootedness

Tomato

Fear-based behavior for any species or breed

Weakness of character

Fear of known origin

Fear of unknown origin

Skittish or easily spooked

Fear of noise or loud voices

Hissing (cats)

Being easily startled

Fear of routine visits to the vet

Trauma of city life

Fear of relocation

Fear of transportation

Fear of kennels, cages, or stalls

Fear of people (adults or children)

Withdrawn from having been bullied

Runt of the litter

Cowering

"Doormat" personality

Excessive fear-based barking

Attacking out of fear

Fear of other animals

Fear of predators

Fear of the outdoors

Fear of new experiences

Need for strengthening

Need for support in guarding or serving people

Plot Qualities and Behaviors of Pet Owners

Almond
Nervousness
Chain-smoking
Compulsive eating
Overwork
Not budgeting enough time for pet
Needing to re-prioritize time
Needing to restore balance
High-strung temperament
Scattered energy
Tension
Living too much through the senses
Sexual excess
Oversleeping
Over-extension of energy
Imbalance

Apple
Worry
Anticipation of problems
Hypochondria
Health-related fears
Doubts
Nagging thoughts
Over-vaccination of one's animals
Over-supplementation of one's pets
Communicating one's own fears to pets
Questioning one's own ability to stay well
Debilitating attitudes
"Doubting Thomas" attitude
Recovering from illness, accidents, or surgery

Avocado

Neglectful pet care

Not spending needed time with pets

Needing to be reminded that pets are a privilege

Forgetting routines for pets

Need for remembrance of the true purpose of having pets

Need to live in the moment

Being "spaced out"

Need for improved focus on pet/owner relationship

Need for mindfulness of the pet's needs

Need for regular attention

Need for mindfully-given love

Banana

Need for humility

Lack of calmness

Quarrelsome attitudes

Inability to recognize one's part in the pet's problems

Pride

Self-defensiveness

Need for admitting to, and learning from, mistakes

Need to administer sensitive discipline

Need to provide higher quality of life for pets

Need to "see the bigger picture"

Easily relinquishing one's pets

Need to listen to one's animals

Unwillingness to admit one's own contributions to pet's problems

Self-protectiveness

Blackberry

Negativity

Unpleasant mental state

Foul temperament

Withdrawal of pets from owner
"Carping spirit"
Pessimism
Unkindness
Meanness of spirit
Verbal cynicism
Sarcasm
Disturbing behaviors for pets
Difficult emotional or psychological issues
Need for clarity
Need to seek insight
Need for rehabilitation of emotional awareness

Cherry
Grumpiness
Moodiness aimed at self
Orneriness
Emotional vacillation
Unnerving attitudes for pets
Mopishness (in pet mirroring the owner)
Unhappiness
Gloom
"Yo-yo" state of mind
Clouding of happiness
Inconsistency in providing discipline
Lack of even-mindedness
Need for detachment in discipline
Apologetic nature
Tyrannical attitudes
Need for help in dealing with an animal's passing

Coconut
"Commitment Essence"
Giving up on one's pet

Abandonment of animals
Perseverance
Need to find answers to pet-related problems
Giving up
Need to "look before leaping" when adoption is considered
Need to learn important lessons
Need for help when pets become problems
Loss of a pet
Need to provide support for animals

Corn
Boredom
Raising lifeless animals
Need to praise one's pets
Need to share excitement
Old attitudes
Inactivity
Listlessness
Need for a "jump start"
Lack of energy
Lack of enthusiasm
Joylessness
Procrastination
Need for exercise
Lethargy
Depression
Beginning a new job
Starting a new school term

Date
Sour disposition
Unwelcoming nature
Lack of hospitality
Unfriendliness

Unmagnetic attitude
Judgmentalism
Lack of acceptance of others
Raising irritable and irritating pets
Lack of charity
Raising fighting, squabbling, hissing, and growling pets
Raising highly territorial pets

Fig
Rigidity
Basic discomfort
Lack of self-acceptance
Unhappiness in one's pets
Overly-corrective nature
Overly-disciplining temperament
Lacking fluidity
Creating an unending series of rules to which pets must conform
Lack of relaxed home atmosphere
Tension-based health problems
Raising jittery pets
Raising animals on edge

Grape
Loneliness
Sense of isolation
Fostering lonely animals
Neglect of pets
Cruelty
Meanness
Sharpness in voice
Abuse of pets
Incompleteness
Lack of love
Death of a spouse

Lack of friends
Loss of a pet
Neediness

Lettuce
Tension
Lack of calmness
Emotional upheaval
Inpatience with pets
Making others jittery
Over-excitement
Discomfort
Inability to express oneself
Inability to share feelings
Poor communication skills
Lack of concentration
"Static in the attic"
Anger
Emotional outbursts
Regret from speaking with anger

Orange
Heaviness
Lack of joy
Lack of hope
Depression
Creating flighty animals
Depression
Lack of lightness
Unhappy emotional climate in home

Peach
Causing problems for pets
Codependence

Conditional love
Need-based pet-owner relationship
Fear of loss
Constant tension
Inability to enjoy one's animals
Over-protectiveness
Fretfulness
Smothering
Being demanding of pets
"Strings attached" love
Over-concern for animals' welfare
Adoption of new animal to replace the old
Unrealistic expectations of a new pet

Pear
"Emergency Essence"
Trauma
Accidents
Illness
Surgeries
Crisis brought on by animal's injuries
"Basket case" state of mind
Off-balance
"Out of sorts"
Quarrelsome nature
Anxiety
Disturbance
Antagonism
Lack of peacefulness
Distressing situations
Visiting relatives
Asking for a raise at work
Lost peace of mind
Upset

A stressful day
Negative influences

Pineapple
Insecurity
Financial worries
Fear of lack of support
Failure to give animal proper supplies
Fear of lack
Fear of not being able to replenish funds
Lack of belief in oneself
Fostering confused animals
Inferiority complex
Drawing to oneself the lack feared
Uncertainty
Taking longer to train pets
Finding regular retraining necessary

Raspberry
Feeling inappropriately responsible for pets
Self-blame
Lack of forgiveness
Grudge-holding
Fiery temper
Unhealed emotional wounds
Bitterness over lost love relationships
Venting frustrations on animals
Harsh speech to pets
Easily relinquishing one's pets
Debarking, declawing, or unnecessarily euthanizing one's pets

Spinach
Stress
Lack of trust

"The classic worrier"
Being overly analytical
Loss of the sense of fun
Dysfunctional childhood
Complicated mental outlook

Strawberry

Loss of one's sense of dignity
Lack of nobility
Sense of undeservedness
Living in a troubled home
Nonsupportive role models
Lack of self-worth
Guilt
Innate worthlessness
Nonproductive attitudes
Self-blaming

Tomato

Fear
Weakness
Fear of known origin
Fear of unknown origin
Feeling overwhelmed by difficulties
Fear of accidents
Fear of flying
Fear of natural disasters
Addictive personality
Tobacco smoking
Overeating
Addiction to unhealthy relationships
Troubled pet behavior
Passing one's own fear to pets

REPERTORIES OF QUALITIES AND BEHAVIORS

This section includes two comprehensive repertories that list both positive and negative qualities and behaviors. It compiles theme essences and plot essences, both pivotal and peripheral. The first repertory applies to animals, the second to people. Some of the essences overlap; hence, addressing the same issue from several angles, the quality of *adaptability* lists Coconut as well as Fig. Also, for clarity, you will find some items listed twice—such as *Confidence, lack of* and *Lack of confidence*.

For the most part, the qualities and behaviors listed here are deliberately not defined by, and thus are not limited to, a species or breed. When you locate the essence for the quality you are seeking, you may refer to that section of the book for a more complete description. Please note: Even when a physical symptom is listed, such as bites, scrapes, or scratches, the remedies address the emotional repercussions of these states and not the injuries themselves. Flower essences do not directly treat physical states or symptoms.

Repertory of Qualities and Behaviors for Animals

Abandonment — Grape
Absorption
   emotions of household — Spinach
   of owner's negativity — Blackberry
Abuse — Orange, Spinach
Acceptable behavior, unsure of — Fig
Acceptance, need for — Fig
Accidents — Pear
Accommodating — Banana
Accommodation of newer energies — Lettuce
Acting older than one's years (when young) — Spinach
Adaptability — Coconut, Fig
Adaptation
   to indoor life — Orange
   to too many rules — Fig
Adjusts well — Grape

Bites	Pear
Biting	Pear
fear-based	Tomato
feeling left out	Grape
jealousy	Grape
vying for attention	Grape
weaning-related	Peach
Bladder control, loss of	Strawberry
Boarding	Pear
Bonding, deep	Raspberry
Boundaries, need for setting comfortable	Cherry
Bowel control, loss of	Strawberry
Breaking existing bad habits, need for	Fig
Bright nature	Coconut
Brooding nature	Spinach
Bruises	Pear
Bullied, withdrawn from having been	Tomato
Bullying, animals who are	Grape
Burns	Pear
Cages, fear of	Tomato
Caginess	Almond
Called, failure to come when	Avocado
Calling (horses)	Pear
Calming effect on others	Pear
Calmness	Almond, Banana, Lettuce
lack of	Almond, Banana
nervous and needing	Pear
Care	
inability to, properly for themselves	Blackberry, Strawberry
poor	Pineapple
-taker	Peach
Cat, bringing home prey	Pineapple
Cautious behavior	Pineapple
Change	
difficulty from	Corn, Pineapple
feeding schedule, in	Pear
home, in the	Fig
ownership, in	Fig
people, positively	Pear
Charm	Pineapple, Strawberry

Cheerfulness	Cherry
Cheerlessness	Cherry
Chemical exposure to, harmful	Blackberry
Chewing	Almond
on furniture or clothing	Peach
Childhood, functional	Apple
Children	
fear of	Tomato
good with	Banana, Peach, Raspberry
living in household with	Pineapple
Clawing as though nursing	Peach
Cleanliness	Blackberry
in soiled or sprayed-on areas	Blackberry
Clinginess	Grape
Comfort	
giving	Lettuce, Raspberry
sense of	Fig, Pear
Commitment	Grape
Communicator, good	Lettuce
Companion	
draws	Date
loss of	Avocado, Grape, Orange
-ship	Banana, Orange
Concern for others' welfare	Peach
Confidence, lack of	Pineapple
Confusion	Fig
by too many rules	Fig
Consistent discipline, lack of	Fig
Constancy	Grape
Contact, eye	Raspberry
Contemplative nature	Lettuce
Contentment	Almond
Contrary behavior	Cherry
Control, in habits	Almond
being out of	Almond
"Couch potato," being a	Corn
Courage	Tomato
Cowering	Tomato
Crabbiness	Date

Crises	Pear
good in	Pear
Curiosity, need to spark	Avocado, Corn
Danger, alerting people to	Tomato
Dangerous behavior	Grape
Dearness	Grape
Death	
loss through	Grape, Orange
nearing	Pear, Strawberry
Debarking	Orange
Declawing	Orange
Delight	Spinach
in abilities and environment	Corn
Demanding	Peach
Demonstrative, overly	Peach
Dependence, emotional	Peach
Depression	Orange
hormonally based	Orange
owners, in	Orange
Despair	Orange
Destruction of property, obsessive	Almond
Devotion	Grape
Difficulty	
facing	Tomato
household, in the	Strawberry
in grooming or caring for self	Strawberry
in training	Strawberry
with change	Corn, Pineapple
Dignity, offended	Strawberry
Disapproval, expressions of	Grape
Discipline	
feels lack of firm, loving, consistent	Fig
reaction to harsh	Raspberry
Disfavor, expressions of	Date
Dislikes, expressions of	Date
Discontentment	Fig
Disorientation	Pear
Distractions, removal of	Lettuce
Disturbance of normal routine	Pear

Divorce of partners	Strawberry
Dog	
guard	Tomato
seeing-eye	Tomato
guarding property	Pineapple
police	Tomato
Domesticated life, stress of	Spinach
Domestication, unnatural altering for	Orange
"Doormat" personality	Tomato
Doubt, owner-caused	Apple
Dreaminess	Avocado
Drooling	Peach
Dysfunctional household, living in	Spinach
Early life, neglect in	Spinach
Easy-going nature	Cherry, Fig
Eating habits, variations in	Fig
Embarrassment with training errors	Strawberry
Embracing nature, an	Date
Emergency Essence	Pear
Emotional	
behavior, overly	Banana
dependence	Peach
-based lack of calmness	Lettuce
struggle	Orange
Emotions, absorbed from household	Spinach
Endurance of illness or injury	Pear
Energy	Corn, Lettuce
lack of	Corn
"reads energy"	Raspberry
unfocused	Avocado
Enjoyment	Orange
lack of	Corn
Entertaining personality	Cherry
Enthusiasm	Corn
Environment, loss of interest in	Spinach
Equilibrium, restoring	Pear
Equanimity	Pear
Errors, embarrassment in training	Strawberry
Even temperament	Cherry
Exercise-wise	Apple

Exhaustion	Corn, Orange
Experiences	
fear of new	Tomato
likes new	Corn
Explore, need to	Corn
Explorer, an	Apple, Avocado
Exposure to harmful chemicals	Blackberry
Expression of preferences	Pineapple, Strawberry
Eyes	
expressive	Raspberry
responsive	Raspberry
Falls	Pear
Fear	
-based behavior	Tomato
health-related through owner	Apple
reinforcement of owner's	Apple
Fearful behavior	Pineapple
Fed by others, needing to be	Strawberry
Feeding	
schedule, changes in	Pear
time, insistence upon	Peach
Feeling	
hurt	Raspberry
nature, a	Raspberry
threatened by younger pets in the household	Peach
Feistiness	Date
Firm discipline, lack of	Fig
Flexibility	Fig
Flowing personality	Fig
Focus, lack of	Avocado, Lettuce
Following owner around	Peach
Food	
intolerance of	Fig
loss of interest	Grape
picky eater	Strawberry
Forgotten, being	Grape
Foster home, raised in a	Pineapple
Frenetic habits	Almond
Friend, lifelong	Grape
Friendliness	Raspberry

Fullness of personality	Grape
Fun	
lack of	Spinach
-loving spirit	Spinach
Furniture, shredding	Raspberry
Fussiness	Fig
Gentleness	Banana
Get along with other pets in the household, need to	Peach
"Getting it," not	Peach
Gnawing themselves or objects	Almond
"Going nuts"	Lettuce
Good	
-natured	Apple, Cherry
with people, especially children	Raspberry
Grace	Strawberry
Grief	Grape, Orange
untouched by	Orange
Grooming	
-conscious	Blackberry
difficulty in	Strawberry
inability to	Blackberry
Grounding, needing	Strawberry
Group participant, a	Banana
Grudge-holding nature	Raspberry
Grumpiness	Cherry
Guard	
animals, for	Tomato
dog	Tomato
Guarding property, dog	Pineapple
Guile, lack of	Blackberry
Happiness	Cherry, Corn, Orange
Harsh discipline, reaction to	Raspberry
"Healer," the	Pear
Health	
consciousness of	Apple
glow of	Apple
-related fears, passed on through owner	Apple
Heat stroke	Pear
High-strung nature	Spinach

Hissing	Raspberry, Tomato
History	
of multiple homes	Orange, Pineapple
unknown past	Fig, Grape, Pear, Tomato
Holds grudges	Raspberry
Honoring of pet's preferences, need for	Cherry
Hormonally-based depression	Orange
Households, living in with other animals	Pineapple
Housing, living in temporary	Pineapple
Humility	Banana
Hurt feelings	Raspberry
Identity	
sense of own	Pineapple
weak sense of	Pineapple
Illness	Pear
battle with terminal	Orange
imminent	Apple
magnified propensity toward	Orange
ongoing	Orange
recovery from	Apple
relapse of	Orange
upsets due to	Pear
Immune system, weakened	Orange
Impending events, barometer of	Pear
Indoors when accustomed to roaming free	Almond
Infancy, healthy	Apple, Grape
Infirmities	
adjustment to	Apple
ongoing physical	Orange
Injury	Orange
pets left overnight at the hospital	Pear
Innocence	Blackberry, Spinach
Inquisitiveness	Avocado
Insecurity	Pineapple
Insensitivity	Raspberry
Insistence on meals before feeding time	Peach
Instability	Pear, Strawberry
Instinctual intelligence	Tomato
Integration	Corn

"Listener," a good	Raspberry
Listlessness	Grape, Orange, Spinach
Loneliness	Grape
Loss	
of bladder or bowel control	Strawberry
of companion	Orange
of interest in environment	Spinach
of interest in food	Grape
of owner or animal friend	Grape
of spirit	Orange
of young	Peach
through death	Orange
through relocation	Orange
Loud voices, fear of	Tomato
Love	Date, Grape, Peach
Loving	
discipline, lack of	Fig
guidelines and parameters, need for	Cherry
Loyalty	Grape
Marking	Grape, Raspberry
Maturity	Avocado, Blackberry, Strawberry
Mean	
-spirited nature	Raspberry
-tempered behavior	Grape
Memory	
of mistreatment	Raspberry
good	Avocado
poor	Avocado
Messages, mixed, from owner	Fig
Mirroring the owner's needs	Cherry
Mistreatment, memory of	Raspberry
Misunderstood	Raspberry
Moderation	
in all habits	Almond
need for	Almond
Moment, lives in	Avocado
Moodiness	Banana, Cherry
Mothering nature	Peach
Move, adjustment after a	Corn

Over-possessiveness	Peach
Overweight	Almond
Owner	
-related problems	Fig, Strawberry
responsiveness to	Avocado
Ownership, changes in	Fig
Owner, depressed	Orange
Pacing (horses)	Pear
Panic	Pear
Patience	Banana
Peace, restoring	Pear
People	
fear of	Tomato
good with, especially children	Raspberry
Peppier, need to be	Corn
Perkier, need to be	Corn
Perseverance	Coconut
Physical	
conditions, ability to deal with difficult	Blackberry
infirmities, ongoing	Orange
Picking on other animals	Date
Picky nature, a	Date
Play, expressing viciousness	Grape, Raspberry
Playfulness	Cherry, Spinach
lack of	Spinach
Poise	Strawberry
Police dog	Tomato
Poor	
care	Pineapple
memory	Avocado
training	Pineapple
Possessiveness, over-	Peach
Posture, upright	Tomato
Praise, appreciation of	Pineapple
Predators, fear of	Tomato
Preferences, expression of	Pineapple, Strawberry
Pregnancy	Orange
Premature weaning	Peach
Presence, strongly felt	Lettuce
Prey, cat bringing home	Pineapple

Pride, genuine, innocent	Pineapple
Propensity toward illness, magnified	Orange
Puncture wounds	Pear
Purity	Blackberry
"Put out to pasture"	Spinach
Quietude	Almond, Lettuce, Strawberry
"Reads energy"	Raspberry
Rearranging furniture, upset from	Corn
Recovery from trauma or surgery	Pear, Spinach
Recuperation time, lengthy	Strawberry
Refinement of character	Strawberry
Reflective personality	Lettuce
Reinforcement of owner's fears	Apple
Relapse of illness	Orange
Relaxation	Fig, Spinach
of territorial instincts	Peach
Relocation	
fear of	Tomato
loss through	Orange
Removal of distraction	Lettuce
Renewed interest in life	Corn
Rescue animal, natural	Tomato
Resentment	Raspberry
toward affection shown to other pets	Raspberry
Resilience	Orange
Responsible nature	Strawberry
Restlessness	Lettuce
Restoration of	
a sense of adventure	Corn
peace and equilibrium	Pear
Retain information, need for the ability to	Avocado
Richness	Cherry, Strawberry
Rigid nature	Fig
Riled, becoming inappropriately	Banana
"Roamer," the	Avocado
Robustness, need for	Apple
Routine	
disturbance of normal	Pear
transportation, fear of	Tomato

variations in established	Fig
visits to the vet, fear of	Tomato
Royalty	Strawberry
Rules, lack of adaptation to too many	Fig
Runt of the litter	Apple, Pineapple, Tomato
"Sadness absorber"	Orange
Saving lives	Tomato
Scent of previous animals, living with	Pineapple
Scrapes	Pear
Seeing-eye dog	Tomato
Self-	
assuredness	Pineapple
involvement	Peach
Selflessness	Peach
Sense of adventure, restoration of	Corn
Sensitivity	Banana, Raspberry
Separation	
of partners	Strawberry
temporary	Peach
Setbacks	Orange
Setting comfortable boundaries, need for	Cherry
Severing ties with people or animals	Grape
Sharing nature, a	Peach
Shock	Pear
Short attention span	Avocado, Lettuce
Shows, taken to	Pineapple
"Show stopper"	Pineapple
Shredding of furniture	Raspberry
Shying away from people	Pineapple
Simplicity	Spinach
Sincere friend, a	Cherry
"Sixth sense"	Tomato
Skittish nature	Tomato
Sleek in appearance	Blackberry
Sleeping habits, variations in	Fig
Slow learning	Avocado
Sluggishness in	
bodily habits	Spinach
the owner	Corn
Soiling	Grape, Raspberry

Soothing personality	Spinach
Sophistication	Avocado, Strawberry
Sour disposition	Date
"Sour puss," being a	Cherry
Specialness	Date
Spoiled	Cherry
Spooked, easily	Tomato
Spraying	Grape, Raspberry
"Spunkiness," loss of	Corn
Stalls, fear of	Tomato
Stamina	Coconut
Startled, easily	Tomato
Steadiness	Pear
Stings	Pear
Stray, having been a	Spinach
Strength	Tomato
Strengthening, need for	Tomato
Stress	Almond, Spinach
-free character	Spinach
living in home with	Spinach
of domesticated life	Spinach
Struggle, emotional	Orange
Suckling furniture or clothing	Peach
Support with allopathic or other medications	Pear
Surface wounds	Pear
Surgeries	Pear
Surgery, recovering from trauma of	Pear, Spinach
Sweetness	Date
Temporarily housed animals	Pineapple
Tenderness	Date
Tension	Lettuce
Terminal illness, battling	Orange
Territorialism	
over- or inappropriate	Grape, Peach
need to relax	Peach
Territory, threatened	Strawberry
"Therapist," the	Blackberry
Threatened, senior pets feeling	Grape, Peach
Training	
embarrassment of errors	Strawberry

incorrect	Fig
need for support in	Avocado, Fig
poor	Pineapple
responsiveness to	Avocado
Transcendence	Coconut
Transportation	Pear
fear of	Tomato
Trauma	Pear
of city life	Tomato
recovery from	Pear, Spinach
Troubled feelings	Cherry
Trusting companion	Blackberry, Peach, Spinach
Unacceptable, feeling his behavior is	Fig
Unapproachableness	Grape
Unassertiveness	Banana
Uncleanliness, sense of	Blackberry
Uncertain of what behavior is acceptable	Fig
Undemanding nature	Almond, Lettuce
Undermined orientation to home or property	Pineapple
Unflappable nature	Pear
Unfocused energy	Avocado
Unforgiving nature	Raspberry
Unhappiness	Orange
Unhealthy	
behavior	Apple
human role model	Blackberry
Unknown	
fears	Tomato
past history	Fig
Unobtrusiveness	Almond
Unresponsiveness	Avocado
Unsupportive home environment	Pineapple
Unsure of self	Fig, Pineapple
Untidiness, offended by	Blackberry
Upliftment	Coconut
Uprootedness	Strawberry
Upset	
from rearranging furniture	Corn
due to illness	Pear

Variations in eating or sleeping habits	Fig
Veterinarian	
visits to	Peach, Pear
fear of routine visits to	Pear, Tomato
Viciousness expressed in play	Grape, Raspberry
Vitality	Corn
Vulnerability, sense of	Apple
Walk, inability to	Strawberry
Weakened immune system	Orange
Weak sense of identity	Pineapple
Weakness, sense of	Apple
Weaning, premature	Peach
Welcoming of life	Tomato
Whininess	Fig
for no apparent reason	Grape
Withdrawn	Tomato
behavior	Grape, Raspberry
behavior after a move	Corn
Worry, owner-induced	Apple
Worth, lack of	Strawberry
Worth-affirming	Strawberry
Wound-up behavior	Lettuce
Wounds, surface or puncture	Pear
Young, acting older than one's years when	Spinach
Young, loss of	Grape, Orange, Peach
Youthful immaturity	Lettuce
Youthfulness	Cherry
Zest, lack of, for new experiences	Corn

Repertory of Qualities and Behaviors for Pet Owners

Abandonment of animals	Coconut
Abused animals, good with previously	Grape
Ability to stay well, questioning own	Apple
Abuse of pets	Grape
Acceptance	Date
of others, lack of	Date
of self	Fig

Accidents	Pear
fear of	Tomato
recovery from	Apple
Activities, enjoyment of children's	Spinach
Adaptability	Fig
Addictive personality	Tomato
Admission	
of, and learning from mistakes	Banana
of mistakes	Banana
of their contribution to pet's problems	Banana
Adoption	
"look before leaping" when considering	Coconut
of another pet when one has passed on	Tomato
of new animals to replace lost ones	Peach
Adored by pets	Orange
Agitation, calming to emotional	Lettuce
Alertness	Avocado
Anger	Lettuce
regret from speaking with	Lettuce
Answers, finding, to pet-related problems	Coconut
Antagonism	Pear
Anticipation of worries	Apple
Anxiety	Pear
Apologetic nature	Cherry
Attention, need for regular	Avocado
Attitudes	
debilitating	Apple
"doubting Thomas"	Apple
nonproductive	Strawberry
old	Corn
tyrannical	Cherry
unmagnetic	Date
unnerving for pets	Cherry
Availability for pets	Almond
Awareness	Coconut
rehabilitation of emotional	Blackberry
Balance	Almond
off	Pear
"Basket case" state of mind	Pear

Beauty	Strawberry
Befriending others	Grape
Behaviors disturbing to pets	Blackberry
Belief in oneself, lack of	Pineapple
Bitterness over lost love relationships	Raspberry
Blends energy with pets	Fig
Bonds with animals	Coconut
Boredom	Corn
"Brave warrior"	Tomato
Breeds irritable and irritating pets	Date
Bubbliness	Cherry
Budgeting too little time for pets	Almond
Calming to the emotionally agitated	Lettuce
Calmness	Almond, Banana, Lettuce
lack of	Lettuce
Care, neglectful pet	Avocado
Caring owner	Raspberry
"Carping spirit"	Blackberry
Causes problems for pets	Peach
Chain-smoker	Almond
Charisma	Pineapple
Charity, lack of	Date
Cheerfulness	Cherry
Childhood	
dysfunctional	Spinach
healthy	Spinach
Childlike nature	Cherry, Spinach
Children's activities, enjoyment of	Spinach
Clarity, need for	Blackberry
"Classic worrier"	Spinach
Cleanliness	Blackberry
Clouding of happiness	Cherry
Codependence	Peach
Comfort	Pear
in different environments	Fig
to pets	Lettuce
Comfortable companion	Almond
"Commitment Essence"	Coconut
Communication	Peach
skills, good	Lettuce

skills, poor	Lettuce
Companion	
comfortable	Almond
empowering	Strawberry
good	Fig
Compassion	Raspberry
Complicated mental outlook	Spinach
Compulsive eater	Almond
Concentration	Avocado
lack of	Lettuce
Concern for others	Peach
Concerned owner	Raspberry
Conditional love	Peach
Conform, to owner's rules	Fig
Confused animals, fosters	Pineapple
Connection with animals	Grape
Consistency of energy	Corn
"Counselor," the	Blackberry
Courage	Tomato
Creative, highly	Lettuce
Crisis brought on by animal's injury	Pear
Cruelty	Grape
Cynicism, verbal	Blackberry
Death	
of a pet	Cherry, Coconut, Grape
of a spouse	Grape
Debilitating attitudes	Apple
Defensiveness, self	Banana
Definite ideas on many issues	Pineapple
Demanding of pets	Peach
Depression	Orange
supportive of owner's	Orange
Detachment in discipline, needs	Cherry
Devotion	Grape
Difficulties	
emotional or psychological	Blackberry
overwhelmed by	Tomato
sustained through	Orange
Dignity	Strawberry
Disasters, fear of natural	Tomato

of children's activities	Spinach
Environments, comfort in different	Fig
Even-mindedness	Cherry
lack of	Cherry
Excellent pet owner	Spinach
Excess, sexual	Almond
Excitement, need to share	Corn
Exercise	Corn
need for	Corn
Expansive nature	Peach
Expectations, unrealistic, of new pet	Peach
Express oneself, unable to	Lettuce
Facilities, improvements on	Corn
Fear	Tomato
communicated and passed on to pets	Apple
health-related	Apple
of flying	Tomato
of known origin	Tomato
of lack	Pineapple
of lack of support	Pineapple
of loss	Peach
of natural disasters	Tomato
of not being able to replenish funds	Pineapple
of unknown origin	Tomato
Fearless animals, breeders of	Tomato
Feelings, cannot share	Lettuce
Fiery-tempered owners	Raspberry
Fighting, a home with	Date
Financial worries	Pineapple
Firm disciplinarian, loving and	Tomato
Flexibility	Fig
Flighty animals, creates	Orange
Fluidity	Fig
lacking	Fig
Flying, fear of	Tomato
Focus on pet/owner relationship, improved	Avocado
Focused mind	Avocado
Forgetting routines for pets	Avocado
Forgiveness	Raspberry
lack of	Raspberry

Forthrightness	Tomato
Foul temperament	Blackberry
Fretting owner	Peach
Friends	
good to talk to	Blackberry
lack of	Grape
makes readily	Date
Frustrations vented on animals	Raspberry
Fullness in energy	Orange
Fun	Spinach
lost sense of	Spinach
-oriented	Cherry
Gallantry	Tomato
Generosity	Strawberry
Gentleness	Banana, Raspberry
Getting along with other household pets	Peach
Giving up	Coconut
on pets	Coconut
Gladness	Orange
Gloom	Cherry
Good	
memory	Avocado
-natured personality	Cherry
with previously abused animals	Grape
Graciousness	Strawberry
Grounding	Strawberry
Growling, a home with	Date
Grudge-holding	Raspberry
Grumpiness	Cherry
Guilt	Strawberry
Happy pets, raises	Orange
Harsh speech to pets	Raspberry
"Health nut"	Apple
Health problems, tension-based	Fig
sensitivity to pet's	Apple
Health-related fears	Apple
Healthfulness	Apple
Healthy childhood	Spinach
Heaviness	Orange
High-strung temperament	Almond

Hissing, a home with	Date
Home	
atmosphere, lack of relaxed	Fig
troubled	Strawberry
unhappy emotional climate in	Orange
with fighting, squabbling, hissing, and growling	Date
"Homebody"	Almond
Honesty	Spinach
Hope, lack of	Orange
Hospitality	Date
lack of	Date
Household, creates unemotional	Banana
shares easily with pets	Banana
Humility	Banana
need for	Banana
Humor, kindly sense of	Blackberry
Hypochondria	Apple
Ideal pet owner	Raspberry
Illness	Pear
recovery from	Apple
Imbalance	Almond
Impatience with pets	Lettuce
Impersonal nature	Banana, Cherry
Improvement	
of facilities	Corn
-oriented	Coconut
Inability to recognize one's part in pet's problems	Banana
Inactivity	Corn
Incompleteness	Grape
Inconsistent disciplinarian	Cherry
Inconspicuousness	Almond
Individualism	Pineapple
Individuality, respects pet's	Pineapple
Inferiority complex	Pineapple
Influences, negative	Blackberry, Pear, Tomato
Informed, nutritionally	Apple
Injuries, crisis brought on by animal's	Pear
Innovative personality	Lettuce
Insecurity	Pineapple
Insight, seeking	Blackberry

Insightfulness	Blackberry
Integration of people with pets	Pear
Interest in learning	Avocado
Intuition	Raspberry, Grape
Irritable pets, breeds	Date
Irritated, not easily	Date
Irritating pets, breeds	Date
Isolation, sense of	Grape
Jittery	
makes others	Lettuce
pets	Fig
Job, beginning new	Corn
Joking nature	Cherry
Joy	Orange
in gathering knowledge	Avocado
lack of	Corn, Cherry, Orange
Judgmentalism	Date
"Jump start," need for	Corn
Kindheartedness	Raspberry
Kindly sense of humor	Blackberry
Knowledge, joy in gathering	Avocado
Knowledgeable pet owner	Avocado
Lack of	
abundance, sense of	Pineapple
acceptance of others	Date
belief in oneself	Pineapple
calmness	Almond, Banana, Lettuce
charity	Date
concentration	Lettuce
energy	Corn
even-mindedness	Cherry
fluidity	Fig
forgiveness	Raspberry
friends	Grape
hope	Orange
hospitality	Date
joy	Orange
lightness	Orange
love	Grape
nobility	Strawberry

peacefulness	Pear
relaxed home atmosphere	Fig
self-absorption	Banana
self-acceptance	Fig
self-worth	Strawberry
support, fears	Pineapple
Laughter	Cherry
Lavishing praise on pets	Strawberry
Learning, interest in	Avocado
Learns	
from mistakes	Banana
from pets	Coconut
needed lessons	Coconut
Lessons, learning needed	Coconut
Lethargy	Corn
"Life of the party"	Pineapple
Life, provide higher quality of, for pets	Banana
Lifeless animals, raising	Corn
Lightheartedness	Cherry
Lightness, lack of	Orange
"Listen to" animals, need to	Banana
Listener, good	Raspberry
Listlessness	Corn
Living too much through the senses	Almond
Loneliness	Grape
Lonely animals, fostering	Grape
Loss	
fear of	Peach
of dignity	Strawberry
of peace of mind	Pear
of pet	Coconut, Grape
of sense of fun	Spinach
Love	Grape
conditional	Peach
lack of	Grape
need for mindfully given	Avocado
"strings attached"	Peach
Loving but firm disciplinarian	Tomato
Meanness	Grape
Mellowness	Pear

productive attitudes	Strawberry
supportive role models	Strawberry
trusting	Spinach
Not upset over animal's problems	Lettuce
Nurturance	Grape, Peach
Nutritionally informed	Apple
Obstacles	
faces	Tomato
works through	Coconut
Off-balance	Pear
Old attitudes	Corn
Openness	Fig
Orneriness	Cherry
Others, concern for	Peach
"Out of sorts"	Pear
Outbursts, emotional	Lettuce
Over-	
concern for animal's welfare	Peach
excitement	Lettuce
extension of energy	Almond
protectiveness	Peach
sleeping	Almond
supplementation of pets	Apple
vaccination of animals	Apple
Overly	
analytical	Spinach
corrective nature	Fig
disciplining temperament	Fig
Overwhelmed by difficulties	Tomato
Overwork	Almond
Owner	
abusive	Grape
boring	Corn
causes problems for pets	Peach
concerned and caring	Raspberry
debarking, declawing, or unnecessarily euthanizing one's pets	Raspberry
easily relinquishing one's pets	Banana, Raspberry
excellent	Spinach
fiery-tempered	Raspberry

Problems
    anticipation of   Apple
    causes for pets   Peach
    inability to recognize one's part in pet's   Banana
    upset over animal's, not   Lettuce
    when pets become   Coconut
Procrastination   Corn
Protectiveness of self   Banana
Psychological issues   Blackberry
Purebreds, owner of   Strawberry
Purity   Blackberry
Quality of life for pets, provides higher   Banana
"Quality time" for pets   Coconut
Quarrelsome attitudes   Banana, Pear
Questions own ability to stay well   Apple
Quietness   Lettuce
Raise at work, asking for   Pineapple, Pear
Raising
    happy pets   Orange
    lifeless animals   Corn
Rambunctious animals, match for   Cherry
Reader of pet's body language   Avocado
Recovery from illness, accidents, or surgery   Apple
Refinement   Strawberry
Refreshing, exuberantly   Pineapple
Regret from speaking with anger   Lettuce
Rehabilitation of emotional awareness   Blackberry
Relates deeply to others   Grape
Relaxation   Banana, Fig
Relinquishing one's pets, easily   Banana
Reminded, needing to be, that pets are a privilege   Avocado
Replenish funds, fear of not being able to   Pineapple
Reprioritize time, helps to   Almond
Respects pet's individuality   Pineapple
Responsible
    inappropriately feeling, for pets   Raspberry
    nature   Strawberry
Restore balance, helps to   Almond
Retiring nature   Lettuce

Retraining necessary	Pineapple
Rigidity	Fig
Role models, non-supportive	Strawberry
Rooted, personality firmly	Pear
Routines for pets, forgetting	Avocado
Rules, unending series of	Fig
"Safe" friend	Date
Scattered energy	Almond
School term, starting new	Corn
Self-	
absorption, lack of	Banana
acceptance	Fig
acceptance, lack of	Fig
assuredness	Pineapple
blame	Raspberry, Strawberry
control	Almond
defensiveness	Banana
protectiveness	Banana
worth, lack of	Strawberry
Selflessness	Peach
Senses, living too much through	Almond
Sensitivity	Raspberry
to animal's needs	Peach
to pet's health needs	Apple
Serviceful quality	Peach
Sexual excess	Almond
Share	
excitement, need to with pets	Corn
home easily with animals	Banana
Sharpness in voice	Grape
Simplicity	Spinach
Smile	Cherry
characteristic	Orange
Smothering	Peach
Solidity	Pear
Sour disposition	Date
"Spaced out" owner	Avocado
Speaking with anger, regret from	Lettuce
Speech harsh to pets	Raspberry
Sports participant	Apple

Spouse, death of	Grape
Squabbling, a home with	Date
Stability	Cherry, Pear
Stamina	Apple, Tomato
"Static in the attic"	Lettuce
Straightforwardness	Blackberry, Spinach
Strength	Tomato
Stress	Spinach
Stressful day, a	Pear
"Strings attached" love	Peach
Supplies, does not give animal proper	Pineapple
Support	
fears lack of	Pineapple
of animals	Coconut
of depressed owner	Orange
Surgeries	Pear
recovery from	Apple
Sustains through difficulties	Orange
Sweetness	Date
Sympathy	Raspberry
Tended, pets well	Peach
Tenderness	Date
Tension	Almond, Lettuce
-based health problems	Fig
constant	Peach
Territorial, highly	Date
Thoughts, nagging	Apple
Time with pet	
not budgeting enough	Almond
not spending enough	Avocado
Training of pets	
non-ambivalent	Blackberry
takes longer	Pineapple
Trauma	Pear
Travelers, good	Fig
Troubled	
home	Strawberry
pet behavior	Tomato
Trustworthiness	Spinach
Tyrannical attitudes	Cherry

Unable to express oneself	Lettuce
Uncertainty	Pineapple
Understanding	Raspberry
of pets	Peach
Undeservedness, sense of	Strawberry
Unemotional household, creates	Banana
Unfriendliness	Date
Unhappiness	Cherry
in pets	Fig
of emotional climate in home	Orange
Unhealed emotional wounds	Raspberry
Unimposing personality	Banana
Unkindness	Blackberry
Unmagnetic attitude	Date
Unnerving attitudes for pets	Cherry
Unpleasant mental state	Blackberry
Unwelcoming nature	Date
Unwillingness to admit contribution to pet's problems	Banana
Upheaval, emotional	Lettuce
Upliftment	Coconut
Upset	Pear
Vacillation, emotional	Cherry
Values animals	Pear
Venting frustrations on animals	Raspberry
Visiting relatives	Pear
Vitality	Corn
Voice, sharpness in	Grape
Weakness	Tomato
Well	
-educated	Blackberry
-tended pets	Peach
Willingness to be wrong	Tomato
Willpower	Tomato
Withdrawn nature of pets from owner	Blackberry
Worries, financial	Pineapple
Worry	Apple
Worthlessness, innate	Strawberry
Wrong, willingness to be	Tomato
Younger pets, good with	Cherry
"Yo-yo" state of mind	Cherry

BIBLIOGRAPHY

Devi, Lila. *The Essential Flower Essence Handbook: Remedies for Inner Well-Being*. San Diego, Calif.: Hay House, 1998.

Fitzpatrick, Sonya, and Patricia Burkhart Smith. *What the Animals Tell Me: Developing Your Innate Telepathic Skills to Understand and Communicate with Your Pets*. New York: Hyperion, 1997.

Heinerman, John. *Natural Pet Cures*. Paramus, N.J.: Prentice Hall, 1998.

Linden, Eugene. *The Parrot's Lament*. New York: Penguin Putnam, 1999.

Lynden, Patricia. "Creature Comforts." *New Age Journal*, March–April 2000, 88–95.

Puotinen, C. J. *The Encyclopedia of Natural Pet Care*. New Canaan, Conn.: Keats Publishing, 1998.

Thomas, Warren D., and Daniel Kaufman. *Dolphin Conferences, Elephant Midwives, and Other Astounding Facts about Animals*. Los Angeles: Jeremy P. Tarcher, 1990.

Walters, J. Donald. *Awaken to Superconsciousness: Meditation for Inner Peace, Intuitive Guidance, and Greater Awareness*. Nevada City, Calif.: Crystal Clarity Publishers, 2000.

Wright, Michael. *The Complete Book of Gardening*. New York: Warner Books, 1980.

Yogananda, Paramhansa. *Autobiography of a Yogi*. New York: The Philosophical Library, 1946. Reprint, Nevada City, Calif.: Crystal Clarity Publishers, 1994.

About the Master's Flower Essences

The Master's Flower Essences is a manufacturing and educational center dedicated to furthering the understanding and knowledge of this special method of herbal therapy. If you would like more information about flower essence products (retail or wholesale) or programs (lectures, seminars, consultations, and a tri-level home-study correspondence course), please write to Master's Flower Essences, 14618 Tyler Foote Road, Nevada City, California 95959, USA; or call (530) 478-7655 or fax (530) 478-7652; for toll-free ordering, call 1-800-347-3639. You can also visit our Web site at *www.mastersessences.com* or e-mail us at *mfe@mastersessences.com*. Lila welcomes and appreciates your animal and people stories, testimonials, and inquiries.

ABOUT THE AUTHOR

Lila Devi (pronounced *lee-lah day-vee*) lives in the rugged high desert country of the Sierra Nevada foothills at Ananda Village in Nevada City, California, with her cats and husband. It was here in 1977 that she developed the Master's Flower Essences, the second oldest essence line in the world today. A lifelong love of people and pets has inspired her collection, over the last twenty-three years, of animal case histories that have provided the foundation for *Flower Essences for Animals*.

Lila lectures extensively both nationally and abroad. She brings an expansive view of plants and animals—expressed through her creation of the flower essences—to her programs, radio shows, and television appearances. Drawing on her skills as a writer of songs, poetry, and plays and on her talent as a musician—vocalist, guitarist, and composer—her classes present a fresh and refreshing approach to Nature and awareness.

A graduate with honors from the University of Michigan at Ann Arbor, Lila majored in English and psychology and also earned a secondary-teaching certificate. Teaching English and running a group home for the developmentally disabled preceded her founding of the Master's Flower Essences. Her first book, *The Essential Flower Essence Handbook*, is available in English and Italian.

OTHER BOOKS FROM
BEYOND WORDS PUBLISHING, INC.

Conversations with Dog

An Uncommon Dogalog of Canine Wisdom
Author: Kate Solisti-Mattelon
$13.95, softcover

    Conversations with Dog is a groundbreaking book in the field of human-animal communication. In a question-and-answer format, this is the first book of its kind to pose questions to dogs and receive answers in return. These answers are not based on what human beings suppose dogs think. Instead, Solisti-Mattelon, a practicing animal communicator, goes straight to the dogs themselves. Most of us who own dogs know they are trying to tell us something, and *Conversations with Dog* breaks through the species barrier to ask dogs what they want to tell all of us.

The Holistic Animal Handbook

A Guidebook to Nutrition, Health, and Communication
Authors: Kate Solisti-Mattelon and Patrice Mattelon
$14.95, softcover

    The Holistic Animal Handbook is the first book to bring together practical information about diet, nutrition, and training with animal communication and emotional balancing techniques. The book is the result of the authors' many years of experience working with companion animals and their people. It includes chapters that explain how to prepare healthy, holistic recipes and Bach Flower Remedies for restoring an animal's emotional balance. There is also a chapter that describes natural techniques for dealing with common behavioral and training problems. The goal of *The Holistic Animal Handbook* is to provide animal guardians with a starting point from which they can foster and practice deeper interspecies communication. Focusing primarily on dogs, cats, and horses but relevant to virtually all animals, the book presents a dual premise: healthy companion animals are better equipped to help the humans they love, just as educated humans are better able to comprehend what their animals are about.

Kinship with the Animals

Authors: Michael Tobias and Kate Solisti-Mattelon

$15.95, softcover

Contributors to *Kinship with the Animals* represent a myriad of countries and traditions. From Jane Goodall illustrating the emergence of her lifelong devotion to animals to Linda Tellington-Jones describing her experiences communicating with animals through touch, the thirty-three stories in *Kinship with the Animals* deconstruct traditional notions of animals by offering a new and insightful vision of animals as conscious beings capable of deep feelings and sophisticated thoughts. The editors have deliberately sought stories that present diverse views of animal awareness and communication.

Animal Talk

Interspecies Telepathic Communication

Author: Penelope Smith

$14.95, softcover

If your animal could speak, what would it say? In *Animal Talk*, Penelope Smith presents effective telepathic communication techniques that can dramatically transform people's relationships with animals on all levels. Her insightful book explains how to solve behavior problems, how to figure out where your animal hurts, how to discover animals' likes and dislikes, and why they do the things they do. Without resorting to magic tricks or wishful thinking, *Animal Talk* teaches you how to open the door to your animal friends' hearts and minds. An entire chapter of this illuminating book is devoted to teaching people how to develop mind-to-mind communication with animals. *Animal Talk* also explores the following topics: freedom, control, and obedience; understanding behavior from an animal's point of view; how to handle upsets between animals; tips on nutrition for healthier pets; and the special relationship between animals and children. There is even a section on how to communicate with fleas and other insects!

When Animals Speak
Lessons, Healings, and Teachings for Humanity
Author: Penelope Smith; Foreword: Michael Roads
$14.95, softcover

This book offers deep, life-changing revelations, communicated directly from the animals. Discover who animals and other forms of life really are; how they understand themselves and others; how they feel about humans and life on Earth; how they choose their paths in life and death; the depth of their spiritual understanding and purposes; and how they can teach, heal, and guide us back to wholeness as physical, mental, emotional, and spiritual beings. Regain the language natively understood by all species. Laugh as you experience other species' refreshing and sometimes startling points of view on living in this world, among humans, and with you.

Dolphin Talk
An Animal Communicator Shares Her Connection
Author: Penelope Smith
$9.95, audiotape

Tales of adventure and communications from the dolphins transport us into the excitement and mystery of our eternal connection with these charismatic marine mammals. Smith shares the dolphin healing journey that enabled her to overcome a lifelong fear of deep water and swim with wild dolphins in the open ocean. Feel the special affection for the human species that the dolphins impart; hear about the merging of dolphin and human consciousness; experience the haunting tones of dolphin "resounding skull bone chanting," creating an opening in the listener's skull to better receive the dolphin's energetic transformations. According to Smith, the dolphins facilitate the weaving of energy matrices of consciousness over our planet, allowing receptive and ready humans to receive the dolphins' pure love throughout their cellular structure and to experience telepathic communication. Feel the dolphins' healing power conveyed through this audiotape, directly by them!

Listening to Wild Dolphins

Learning Their Secrets for Living with Joy
Author: Bobbie Sandoz
$14.95, softcover

    Listening to Wild Dolphins, written by a well-established therapist, chronicles her remarkable and healing experiences while swimming with a pod of wild dolphins off the shores of her Hawaiian home over the past ten years. She has observed that the dolphins have qualities which humans can model to become more balanced and joyful in everyday life.

Sacred Flowers

Creating a Heavenly Garden
Author: Roni Jay
$14.95, hardcover

    For thousands of years the magical qualities of flowers have been held sacred by traditions around the world: the lily to the Christian church, the lotus to Asian cultures, the rose to both the Christian and Muslim faiths. *Sacred Flowers* explores the special powers attributed to a fragrant collection of flora. You will discover which flower placed under a pillow can give romantic dreams, which flowering herb will help restore a friendship, which flower pinned to your clothing will protect you, which blossom is an aid to astral projection and prophecy, and which flower will give you the courage to realize your dreams. *Sacred Flowers* reveals the healing properties of flowers for the mind, body, and spirit. You can draw upon this wealth of ancient lore to explore the medicinal or inspirational effects of a fragrance, and the book will help you to design and create a mystical and spiritual paradise in your own yard or patio.

The Great Wing

A *Parable*

Author: Louis A. Tartaglia, M.D.; Foreword: Father Angelo Scolozzi

$14.95, hardcover

The Great Wing transforms the timeless miracle of the migration of a flock of geese into a parable for the modern age. It recounts a young goose's own reluctant but steady transformation from gangly fledgling to Grand Goose and his triumph over the turmoils of his soul and the buffeting of a mighty Atlantic storm. In *The Great Wing*, our potential as individuals is affirmed, as is the power of group prayer, or the "Flock Mind." As we make the journey with this goose and his flock, we rediscover that we tie our own potential into the power of the common good by way of attributes such as honesty, hope, courage, trust, perseverance, spirituality, and service. The young goose's trials and tribulations, as well as his triumph, are our own.

Forgiveness

The Greatest Healer of All

Author: Gerald G. Jampolsky, M.D.; Foreword: Neale Donald Walsch

$12.95, softcover

Forgiveness: The Greatest Healer of All is written in simple, down-to-earth language. It explains why so many of us find it difficult to forgive and why holding on to grievances is really a decision to suffer. The book describes what causes us to be unforgiving and how our minds work to justify this. It goes on to point out the toxic side effects of being unforgiving and the havoc it can play on our bodies and on our lives. But above all, it leads us to the vast benefits of forgiving.

The author shares powerful stories that open our hearts to the miracles which can take place when we truly believe that no one needs to be excluded from our love. Sprinkled throughout the book are Forgiveness Reminders that may be used as daily affirmations supporting a new life free of past grievances.

Teach Only Love

The Twelve Principles of Attitudinal Healing
Author: Gerald G. Jampolsky, M.D.
$12.95, softcover

From best-selling author Dr. Gerald Jampolsky comes a revised and expanded version of one of his classic works, based on A *Course in Miracles.* In 1975, Dr. Jampolsky founded the Center for Attitudinal Healing, a place where children and adults with life-threatening illnesses could practice peace of mind as an instrument of spiritual transformation and inner healing—practices that soon evolved into an approach to life with profound benefits for everyone. This book explains the twelve principles developed at the Center, all of which are based on the healing power of love, forgiveness, and oneness. They provide a powerful guide that allows all of us to heal our relationships and bring peace and harmony to every aspect of our lives.

Every Day God

Heart to Heart with the Divine
Authors: David and Takeko Hose
$14.95, softcover

When Takeko Hose was accidentally shot and paralyzed from the knees down, she and her husband, David, reached out desperately for divine assistance through a succession of what David calls "naked prayers." *Every Day God* is the record of a remarkable communication between authors David and Takeko and God. Not a stickler for ritual, a lofty voice from beyond, or an enigma, their God is a warm and caring parent, eager to nurture and love unconditionally all of His children. Comforting and enlightening, the teachings in *Every Day God* are lighthearted, often humorous, and relevant to modern life. And at the core of each teaching is an invitation to meet this largely undiscovered self within our innermost hearts, a self that flows from our divine source.

The Woman's Book of Dreams
Dreaming as a Spiritual Practice
Author: Connie Cockrell Kaplan; Foreword: Jamie Sams
$14.95, softcover

Dreams are the windows to your future and the catalysts to bringing the new and creative into your life. Everyone dreams. Understanding the power of dreaming helps you achieve your greatest potential with ease. *The Woman's Book of Dreams* emphasizes the uniqueness of women's dreaming and shows the reader how to dream with intention, clarity, and focus. In addition, this book will teach you how to recognize the thirteen types of dreams, how your monthly cycles affect your dreaming, how the moon's position in the sky and its relationship to your astrological chart determine your dreaming, and how to track your dreams and create a personal map of your dreaming patterns. Connie Kaplan guides you through an ancient woman's group form called dream circle—a sacred space in which to share dreams with others on a regular basis. Dream circle allows you to experience life's mystery by connecting with other dreamers. It shows you that through dreaming together with your circle, you create the reality in which you live. It is time for you to recognize the power of dreams and to put yours into action. This book will inspire you to do all that—and more.

Tibetan Wisdom for Western Life
Authors: Joseph Arpaia, M.D., and Lobsang Rapgay, Ph.D.
Foreword: His Holiness the Dalai Lama
$14.95, softcover

By relating meditative practices to specific mental qualities, this book makes meditation a thorough and logical system of personal development. Part I of the book describes the basic practices of centering, attending, concentrating, and opening and how you develop the five mental qualities of Steadiness, Pliancy, Warmth, Clarity, and Spaciousness. Part II describes how to use the practices from Part I to enhance health, performance, relationships, and spirituality in just fifteen minutes per day. The book uses numerous stories and examples of two people, Brian and Maria, to illustrate the techniques. Brian and Maria are amalgams of the hundreds of people the authors have taught, and the inner details of their experience will capture the reader's interest and augment the instructions for the techniques. This is above all a practical book, with a philosophical depth that does not inhibit the reader. The techniques presented are based on a profound wisdom that is expressed in purely Western terms. The presentation is secular as well, so that readers of all traditions will be able to benefit.

Healing Your Rift with God
A *Guide to Spiritual Renewal and Ultimate Healing*
Author: Paul Sibcy
$14.95, softcover

God, says Paul Sibcy, is everything that is. All of us—faithful seekers or otherwise—have some area of confusion, hurt, or denial around this word, or our personal concept of God, that keeps us from a full expression of our spirituality. *Healing Your Rift with God* is a guidebook for finding our own personal rifts with God and healing them. Sibcy explains the nature of a spiritual rift, how this wound can impair our lives, and how such a wound may be healed by the earnest seeker, with or without help from a counselor or teacher. *Healing Your Rift with God* will also assist those in the helping professions who wish to facilitate what the author calls ultimate healing. The book includes many personal stories from the author's life, teaching, and counseling work, and its warm narrative tone creates an intimate author–reader relationship that inspires the healing process.

Divine Intervention

A Journey from Chaos to Clarity

Author: Susan Anderson

Foreword: David Lukoff, Ph.D.; Afterword: Emma Bragdon, Ph.D.

$13.95, softcover

Divine Intervention is a powerfully written and engaging story of spiritual transformation. Susan Anderson's journey from chaos to clarity provides hope and inspiration for anyone facing the challenge of a major crisis or life change. Susan's spiritual emergency causes her to reconnect with her true self and experience an authentic sense of fulfillment and joy that could only be created by a Divine Intervention. Having received rave reviews from doctors, spiritual leaders, and lay readers, this book is a treasure of insight and wisdom that will empower women and men to take charge of their lives. For those wanting to help anyone in a spiritual emergency, also included is a guide and resource directory by Emma Bragdon, Ph.D., author of *Sourcebook for Helping People in Spiritual Emergency*.

The Intuitive Way

A Guide to Living from Inner Wisdom

Author: Penney Peirce; Foreword: Carol Adrienne

$16.95, softcover

When intuition is in full bloom, life takes on a magical, effortless quality; your world is suddenly full of synchronicities, creative insights, and abundant knowledge just for the asking. *The Intuitive Way* shows you how to enter that state of perceptual aliveness and integrate it into daily life to achieve greater natural flow through an easy-to-understand, ten-step course. Author Penney Peirce synthesizes teachings from psychology, East-West philosophy, religion, metaphysics, and business. In simple and direct language, Peirce describes the intuitive process as a new way of life and demonstrates many practical applications from speeding decision making to expanding personal growth. Whether you're just beginning to search for a richer, fuller life experience or are looking for more subtle, sophisticated insights about your spiritual path, The Intuitive Way will be your companion as you progress through the stages of intuition development.

To order or to request a catalog, contact
Beyond Words Publishing, Inc.
20827 N.W. Cornell Road, Suite 500
Hillsboro, OR 97124-9808
503-531-8700 or 1-800-284-9673

You can also visit our Web site at *www.beyondword.com*
or e-mail us at *info@beyondword.com*.

Beyond Words Publishing, Inc.

Our Corporate Mission:

Inspire to Integrity

Our Declared Values:

We give to all of life as life has given us.
We honor all relationships.
Trust and stewardship are integral to fulfilling dreams.
Collaboration is essential to create miracles.
Creativity and aesthetics nourish the soul.
Unlimited thinking is fundamental.
Living your passion is vital.
Joy and humor open our hearts to growth.
It is important to remind ourselves of love.